Oklahoma Notes

Basic-Sciences Review for Medical Licensure
Developed at
The University of Oklahoma, College of Medicine

Suitable Reviews for:
National Board of Medical Examiners (NBME), Part I
Medical Sciences Knowledge Profile (MSKP)
Foreign Medical Graduate Examination in the Medical Sciences (FMGEMS)
Federation Licensing Examination (FLEX)

Oklahoma Notes

Study Skills and Test-Taking Strategies for Medical Students

Find and Use Your Personal Learning Style

Deborah D. Shain

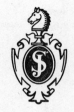

Springer-Verlag

New York Berlin Heidelberg London Paris
Tokyo Hong Kong Barcelona Budapest

Deborah D. Shain
Medical Education Consultant
419 Chapel Road
Elkins Park, PA 19117
USA

Material on pages 4 – 6 was reproduced by special permission of the Publisher, Consulting Psychologists Press, Inc., Palo Alto, CA 94306, from Myers Briggs Type Indicator by Isabel Briggs Myers & Katherine C. Briggs © 1976, 1988. Further reproduction is prohibited without the Publisher's consent.

Library of Congress Cataloging-in-Publication Data
Shain, Deborah D.
    Study skills and test-taking strategies for medical students:
find and use your personal learning style / Deborah D.
Shain.
        p.   cm.
    Includes bibliographical references.
    ISBN 0-387-97695-7
    1. Medicine—Examinations—Study guides.   2. Test-taking skills.
3. Medicine—Study and teaching.   4. Study, Method of.   I. Title.
    [DNLM: 1. Education, Medical.   2. Educational Measurement.
3. Learning.   W 18 S526m]
R834.5.S52   1991
610'.71' 1—dc20
DNLM/DLC
For Library of Congress   91-5150

Camera-ready copy prepared by the author.
Printed and bound by BookCrafters, Chelsea, MI.
Printed in the United States of America.

9 8 7 6 5 4 3 2 1

ISBN 0-387-97695-7 Springer-Verlag New York Berlin Heidelberg
ISBN 3-540-97695-7 Springer-Verlag Berlin Heidelberg New York

Preface

This book, *Study Skills and Test-Taking Strategies for Medical Students: Find and Use Your Personal Learning Style,* is written for the talented medical students who were excellent scholars in undergraduate school but find themselves overwhelmed with the information explosion and time constraints of medical school. Unlike other study-methods books that simply tell what and how to study, this one provides study skills and test-taking strategies that are tailored to fit the learning styles of student, teacher, and practitioner. Knowing how you think, how you process information, how you make decisions, and how you tend to react to your environment will improve your ability to integrate information and to communicate with colleagues and patients.

Medical students have demonstrated that they are sufficiently talented to cope with the rigors of medical school, but many students have discovered that when they study and take exams in medical school, they may appear less competent than they did in college or in other graduate programs.

Study and test-taking strategies developed in undergraduate school, such as multiple readings or rote memorization, do not facilitate the long-term retention and problem-solving abilities required for the practice of medicine. Exams and basic science courses in medical school are different from those given in other settings.

Medical school courses are constructed by many different lecturers, who team-teach loosely organized courses. Students are responsible for the integration of the courses.

The tests require the student to expand study beyond mere understanding and simple recall to knowledge integration, and to the application of that knowledge to a problem-solving situation. The computer-graded, multiple-choice, and true/false exam questions in medical school can be frustrating for both students and their professors. If an examinee misses part of a question, no credit is given for the part that was correct.

Medical schools spend much effort in researching what should be studied and learned, but rarely do they help students achieve the skills to manage the vast amount of material that must be mastered. The information that must be integrated before a physician can practice responsibly can seem endless.

Without a systematic method for organizing the information explosion inherent in the profession of medicine, staying current can be an impossible feat. There is simply too much to learn in the time allotted. The tasks of information management begin in medical school. The techniques offered in this book identify and apply the student's personal learning style to specific methods for study skills and exam-taking strategies so that understanding, analysis, synthesis, and recall of information occur in a time-efficient manner.

The theoretical basis of this method is founded in the work of many scholars of human behavior including Freud, Piaget, Spitz, Mahler, Jung, Briggs, Myers, and McCaulley. Carl Jung's work in psychology revealed that people tend to use certain patterns of interacting in the world. He observed differences in methods of perception and decision-making that people use when working alone and when interacting with others. From his observations, Jung organized a typology. Building on Jung's observations, Katherine C. Briggs and, later, Isabel Briggs Myers expanded and developed type theory.

Based on more than 50 years of research, they developed from their typology, an instrument--the Myers Briggs Type Indicator--that would later be applied to team building in business and family interactions, to methods of education, and then specifically to the health professions.

Myers was particularly interested in students in the health professions because she believed that "accurate perception and informed judgement are especially important in professionals who have other's lives in their hands." The early work was tested with a group of 5355 students of the George Washington School of Medicine. The longitudinal study--of medical students' achievement, drop out rate, and specialty choices--was presented at the American Psychological Association convention in 1964. Mary H. McCaulley developed the work further and went on to study the relationship between type, specialty choices, and professional satisfaction.

Gordon Lawrence, David Keirsey, Marilyn Bates, and researchers of the Association of Psychological Type have conducted studies in family interactions, educational settings, industry, and the health professions. The Shain Method: The Application of Learning-Style-Specific Study Skills and Test-Taking Strategies, developed from 1980 until the present, builds on that research to apply techniques of learning-style-specific study skills and test-taking strategies in medical education.

The methods presented in this book are based on 10 years of classroom-tested workshops and individual tutorials with medical students in the United States, Mexico, and Puerto Rico. As a result of the application and reinforcement of these methods, students, faculty, and administrators report an improvement in students' scores on standardized examinations, classroom tests, essays, and problem-solving exercises.

Acknowledgments

Throughout my 15 years as a medical educator working with students and faculty of medical schools in the United States, Mexico, and Puerto Rico, as I taught, I learned. This book is the result of that teaching and learning process. There are some people without whom this endeavor would have been impossible. To Dr. Richard M. Hyde and his Board Review faculty at the University of Oklahoma Medical School, who began this process, many thanks for your challenge, support, and generosity.

To Dr. Ricardo Leon, the Group Four Faculty, and students of the Universidad Autonoma de Guadalajara Medical School, thanks for contributing to the work and proving that it is effective. To Dr. Sandra Wall and the students and faculty of Meharry Medical College, to Dr. Moses K. Woode of University of Virginia Medical School, to Dr. Joseph O'Donnell of Dartmouth Medical School, to Dr. Fannie E. Brown of University of Tennessee Memphis Medical School, to Carl Ealy of Hahnemann Medical College, to Dr. William Friedman and my mentors at the Fielding Institute, to my fellow researchers in the Association for Psychological Type, to the Health Career Opportunity Program of Bryn Mawr College, and especially to the students and graduates of the Medical College of Pennsylvania who allowed me to enter their lives as they entered their studies, thanks for the impetus and the opportunity to create this method and test its results.

To Dr. Selma Kramer of Jefferson Medical College, for inspiration, friendship and faith, and to Marjorie Shain Horvitz for her gentle and deft hand at editing and surgically shaping the work, thanks for making the book possible.

x

To my friends Ernest and James Witkin, Rina and Newt Malerman, Rita and Bertram Werner, Bernice Rowe, and Pat Dressler, thanks for your hands-on wisdom and loyalty.

To my children by choice, Karen Shain Schloss and Andrew Schloss, thanks for feeding my mind and body. And to all the others of my supportive family-- my late husband, Daniel Shain, my parents, Sybil and Leo Goldstein, my loving children: Martin and Sallie Klein, Scott and Linda Klein, Amy and Daniel Zeff, and energy-restoring grandchildren, and especially to my husband and devoted critic, Morton H. Lerner, without whom I would have been impossible--many thanks beyond work and words.

Contents

xv

CHAPTER ONE • LEARNING STYLES

Have you ever felt frustrated about the results you get on exams? You study hard, but your test scores do not reflect the amount of work you put in. You may have noticed that some colleagues seem to know what to study, put in less work than you, and get better results. The difference may be in the way you have been using your personal *learning style*. Psychological studies have demonstrated that success can depend on your awareness of the methods you use to take in information and how you decide what to do with the information you have studied (Provost and Anchors, 1987).

People differ in how they view the world, how they take in information, and how they take action based on their perceptions. These differences are based on inborn gifts of the mind. Where people tend to focus their attention forms a pattern defined as *psychological type* (Jung, 1923).

Psychological type combined with certain sensory characteristics identified by learning theorists can be classified as a *learning style.* How you use your learning style affects your ability to study efficiently and to achieve success in taking exams (Fratzka, 1989).

Purpose

The purpose of this chapter is to help you identify your personal *learning style* and apply it to specific study and test-taking techniques. You will use your learning style to target study strategies, to determine an environment that will enhance your learning, to help you to achieve higher grades on examinations, and to improve communication skills within a medical team.

Taking Control of the Examination Process

Examination success is directly related to two major factors: the examination and the examinee. In taking a standardized examination, you have no control over the content or form. But what about the examinee? Can you take control of yourself? You can if you know how to identify your limitations and make the most of your talents.

As an academic instrument, you will be able to stay in tune if you discover who you are when you study and who you are when you demonstrate the results of your study efforts. Based on your individual learning style, your grades can improve if you use learning-style-specific techniques for taking in information and making decisions about that information (Shain and Kelliher, 1988).

How do you take in information and make decisions about that information? What is your personal learning style? You can find out by answering a series of questions. The questions you will answer are based on the Myers-Briggs Type Indicator (Myers and McCaulley, 1985), a widely used psychological instrument based on the work of Carl Jung.

In responding to the questions, you will choose between two equally right answers. Your answers will form a pattern revealing your "personality type" and preferred learning style. Once you have answered the questionnaire that follows, your learning style will be represented with a four-letter shorthand coding system. We will then apply that four-letter code to specific study techniques.

The techniques that you have used in the past in other academic settings may work in some subjects but not in others. Once you learn to apply a comprehensive and systematic method of taking in information and deciding what to do with that information, your expanded learning style repertoire can make a significant difference in your grades in all medical school subjects (Leon and Martinez, 1989).

When you are perceiving, amassing, analyzing, and retaining information, and when you are making decisions about that information, what do you prefer to do? What are your favorite study methods?

As you answer these questions, respond in a way that reflects *you* and not someone you think others want you to be. Because there are no right or wrong answers, you may find answering the questions a challenge because both answers are equally attractive. Select the one that seems to appeal to you more *at this time*.

To get yourself in the proper mood for answering the questions, imagine yourself in some comfortable setting. You are on a beach or beside a stream. You are relaxed. Your mind drifts wherever it wants to go. You've kicked your shoes off, and you are thinking about yourself. You wonder, "What makes me tick?"

With a sense of appreciation for who you are, in order to identify aspects of your learning style, please answer the questions of the following pages.

LEARNING STYLE QUESTIONNAIRE

1. If you were a teacher, would you rather teach

   A) fact courses, or

   B) courses involving theory?   A B

2. Do you usually get along better with

   A) realistic people, or

   B) imaginative people?   A B

3. Would you rather be considered

   A) a practical person, or

   B) an ingenious person?   A B

4. Do you admire more the people who are

   A) conventional enough never to make themselves conspicuous, or

   B) too original and individual to care whether they are conspicuous or not?   A B

5. Is it higher praise to say someone has

   A) common sense, or

   B) vision?   A B

6. Do you think it is more important to be able to

   A) adjust to the facts as they are, or

   B) see the possibilities in a situation?   A B

7. Would you rather

   A) go along with the established methods of doing well, or

   B) analyze what is still wrong and attack unsolved problems?   A B

Based on their meaning, not their sound, which word in the following word pairs appeals to you more?

8. A) Facts

    B) Ideas   A B

9. A) Realistic

    B) Speculative   A B

10. A) Literal

    B) Figurative   A B

11. A) Matter-of-fact

    B) Imaginative   A B

12. A) Organized

    B) Spontaneous   A B

13. A) Plan

    B) Discover   A B

Now back to a series of sentences. Please select your preference for A or B.

14. When you have a deadline, do you depend on

    A) starting early, so as to finish with time to spare, or

    B) the extra speed you develop at the last minute?   A B

15. Is it harder for you to adapt to

    A) constant change, or

    B) routine?   A B

16. Do you tend to

    A) make decisions quickly, or

    B) think about many alternatives before deciding?   A B

17. In choosing an answer for a test question, do you tend to

    A) stay with your first decision, or

    B) go back and change your answers?   A   B

18. When studying, do you usually tend to

    A) study just enough, or

    B) feel as though there is much more that you didn't get to?   A   B

19. When it is settled well in advance that you will do something at a certain time,

    do you find it

    A) comforting to be able to plan accordingly, or

    B) a little unpleasant to be tied down?   A   B

20. If you were asked on a Sunday morning, "What you are going to

    do today?" would you

    A) be able to tell with reasonable certainty, or

    B) have to wait to see?   A   B

21. Do you tend to prefer   A   B

    A) closure and the settling of things, or

    B) keeping options open so you can go with the flow?

Now that you have answered the questions, please count the number of A or B
answers in questions 1 through 11, and record them below.

               A_____B_____

In questions 1 through 11, the A answers represent a choice that reflects your
preference for a *mental function* called **Sensing (S)**. The B answers represent your
preference for a *mental function* called **Intuition (N)**.

Mental function? Put simply, a mental function describes how you "tick" when you are perceiving and acting on all of the information in the world. Your preferred mental function reflects how your mind works when it takes in information.

Now count the number of A or B answers in questions 12 through 21 and record them below.

A_____B_____

In questions 12 through 21, the answers represent your attitude about making decisions. The A answers to questions 12 through 21 represent your **Judging (J)** attitude. B answers to questions 12 through 21 represent your **Perceiving (P)** attitude.

Now let's find out what the results mean in terms of your application to study and exam-taking techniques. We'll start with **Sensing (S)** and **Intuition (N)**. You have identified your preferences for attending to *details* **(S)** or enjoying *concepts* **(N)**.

Sensing (S)

If you prefer **Sensing (S)**, you will like subjects that have to do with things you can see, hear, touch, and experience with your five senses. You tend to stay focused in the present, the here and now of what you study. You are interested in what *actually* happened, not what *might* happen.

You would describe yourself as practical, and are firmly grounded in reality. You don't mind routine. When looking at a structure in anatomy, you will notice every detail and the relationship of one detail to another. You appreciate teachers who are organized and follow a sequential format when they lecture.

In your life outside medical school, if you have a mechanical job to do--for example, putting a bike together--you will read the directions *before* you start to assemble the bike. Once you understand the directions, you will proceed step by step and put the bike together. **Sensors** read directions.

Intuition (N)

If your score came out on the **Intuitive (N)** side, you like subjects that allow you to create theories. Physiology is fun because the concepts of physiology permit you to extrapolate results in terms of cause and effect. Ideas and hypotheses fascinate you. You look at patterns rather than specific details. Routine bores you. You would describe yourself as innovative. You tend to be future oriented.

For instance, if, in anatomy, you are presented with a structure, you will probably ask yourself, "What would happen if the structure should happen to change?" You don't mind if teachers digress when they lecture, especially if they provide analogies to illustrate the points that they are trying to make. You think of the lens of the eye as a camera, the heart as a pump.

In your life outside medical school, using the same bike example we used before: When *you* have the bike to put together, you will look at the parts. You will figure out how you *think* it should go together, and start to assemble the little bugger. Once you are finished, if there happen to be parts left over, or if you have had to struggle too much, then you may look at the directions for assembling the bike. **Intuitives** tend to ignore directions. The differences between the way **Sensors** and **Intuitives** perceive the world illustrate the differences you bring with you when you study and take tests.

Sensing types tend to prefer subjects in which "what you see is what you get." Given a structure, S 's will notice the details of the structure, will observe the relationship of one structure to another. Because they use their five senses to take in information, S 's tend to perform very well in recall of details. They work steadily, using "perspiration" to accomplish their perceiving functions.

People who prefer **Intuition,** N's, may not be conscious of noticing the particular details of the structure. They tend to scan and glance. Looking at the whole picture and noting the relationships will give them the clues they will use to extrapolate information about the structure. N 's observe a structure, and then they tend to anticipate immediately the function and the mechanism of action of that structure. They work in spurts, using "inspiration" to accomplish information gathering.

Although we all use both our **Sensing** and our **Intuitive** mental functions, we are inclined to *prefer* either one or the other. All other differences of nature/nurture aside, it is most often our variance in mental function preference that creates the difference in the way different people perceive the same information.

These differences will determine how you, as an S or an N, focus your attention while studying. Different types will tend to anticipate exam questions based on their preferred methods of taking in information. As a result, you will be strong in answering questions that match your learning style, but you may overlook areas that are foreign to your way of taking in information. The trick is to continue to excel in your preferred method, which, because you prefer it, you do well naturally. After all, you have developed that method throughout your life.

Your job now is to develop the less preferred areas, which you might, in the past, have tended to avoid. When you set out to develop your least developed mental function, you may feel slightly uncomfortable. You have little practice in this area, so you may need to be more deliberate as you proceed.

To demonstrate this phenomenon, please follow along with me.
In the space below, using your dominant hand, please write your name as if you were signing it on a check.

_____

Good! That was easy and natural, wasn't it?
Now switch the pencil to your nondominant hand, and sign your name again.

_____

How did that feel? Some students say they feel dumb writing their name with their nondominant hand. They say they feel awkward, silly, childlike, sloppy, and unsettled. That switch from dominant to nondominant hand demonstrates how you will feel when you use the mental function that is not your preferred, or dominant, function.

So if you prefer **Sensing** (S)--that is, you enjoy using your five senses in the here and now--you will feel awkward when you are challenged to take in information that requires you to ask "What would happen if. . . ?" questions.

If you prefer **Intuition** (N)--that is, you enjoy concepts, hypothesizing about the information you tackle--you will feel uneasy when you are asked to restrict your focus to "merely the facts."

To demonstrate the application of your preferred mental function in actual comprehension of medical subjects, let's look at the structure below to see how you take in information about it. This will help you to understand how you put together information in micro and gross anatomy courses involving physical objects.

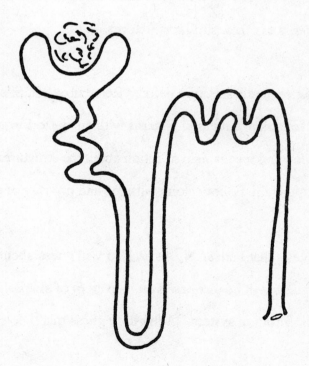

Obviously, this is a diagrammatic representation of a nephron.

If you are a **Sensing** type, you know the parts of the structure well. You have observed the size, shape, color, and number of parts and their relationship to one another. You will be orderly and methodical in your analysis of the structure.

If you are an **Intuitive** type, you will immediately notice the shapes and patterns. You note the differences between the collecting areas, the wiggly areas, the loop, and the straight regions. Your eyes will dart from area to area. You will tend to work in spurts, following your inspiration and curiosity about the entire structure.

Both types notice the relationships of the parts, but the relationships will be perceived with a different focus in mind. For S 's, relationships are seen sequentially. For N 's, relationships are valuable mainly for the formulation of "What would happen if...?" questions and hypotheses. N 's notice similarities within this structure and look for likeness of this structure to the patterns of other, similar structures.

What if you had never seen this structure before? Remember that S 's will look at the details, whereas N's tend to look at structural patterns with an eye to formulating a hypothesis about the function and mechanism of action about the structure. N 's will tend to draw analogies. So look at it again. Follow along with me and my way of perceiving.

My questionnaire reveals that I am an N. As an N, I will guess about the structures I see for the first time. My guess will be that based on its pattern of shapes. I will say, "This thing must be some kind of filtration system." Why did I guess that?

Look at the first part.

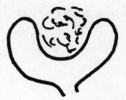

What does it *look like*? What is it *analogous* to? It resembles a funnel, which I have used in the kitchen. Therefore, I guess that it must be the collection area of the structure. Is that right?

Now the next section, the convoluted tube.

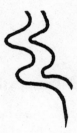

My *association* to the shape of this part of the structure is the route I take when I try to slow myself down while driving on ice, or while skiing down a hill. Why would we want fluid to slow down while passing through this area? Perhaps for reabsorption?

Now the loop area.

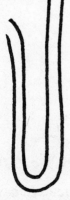

What happens to the fluid when it goes through this area? My guess (*hypothesis*) would be that the pressure of the fluid going down has some relationship to the fluid moving into the upward area. There must be a chemical transfer of something into something else when the fluid moves into the upward section of the tube. Am I right? What *does* happen? Please write your answer in the space below.

Now another convoluted area.

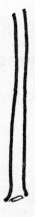

More slowdown; therefore another area of reabsorption? Perhaps there is a difference in the composition of the fluid in this section from the first "slowdown" area? What is that difference?

Now the last section.

It goes straight down. That means that the fluid will travel more quickly than it did through the wiggly areas. So whatever happened before must have finished its chemical transfer and is discharging. Is that right?

If you, too, are an **Intuitive (N)** type, it is natural for you to assume that structure informs function and dictates the process of the mechanism of action. Whereas if you are **a Sensing (S)** type, your eye will pick up every detail. You will see the relationship of one detail to another. But it may not be natural for you to allow yourself to use analogies to everyday life to formulate hypotheses about the function or the mechanism of action regarding an unfamiliar structure found in the human body.

Remember that **Sensing** types stay carefully focused in the here and now, whereas **Intuitive** types tend to jump ahead to "What would happen if. . . ?" questions. The challenge is to do both in order to increase your skills at perceiving all of the available information.

The example above demonstrates learning-style-specific techniques used in understanding *physical objects* courses, such as gross anatomy, embryology, histology, and cell biology.

What methods should you use in the *process* courses, such as physiology, biochemistry, pharmacology, and pathology? Your learning-style strengths will provide you with help as you approach these courses.

Again, you will need to develop strengths in your least preferred mental function. If you prefer **Sensing**, you will need to develop *concepts*. If you prefer **Intuition**, you will need to pay attention to *details*.

In order to demonstrate the use of **Sensing (S)** and **Intuition (N)** mental functions, let's look at the process of protein synthesis that follows.

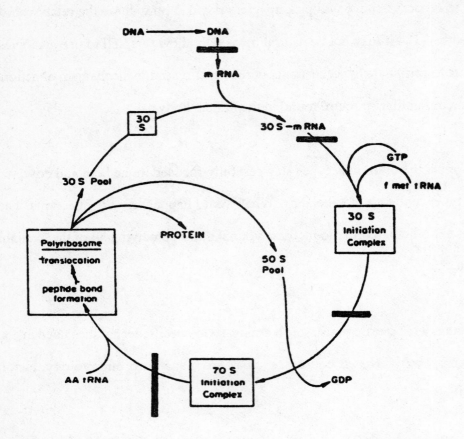

This process, taken from page 20 of the Oklahoma Notes, *Microbiology and Immunology*, depicts a "What would happen if?" situation, in which various antibiotics interfere with protein synthesis. Look again. Notice that there are discrete *steps* to the process. There is a *direction* to the process. There are *requirements* necessary for the process to go from one point to another. There are *inhibitors* to the process.

As you study any process, look for and label: *steps, requirements, changes in direction, coalescence, inhibitors,* and *results* in terms of *cause and effect.* This matrix of study points will apply to any and all subjects that involve process information.

Let's practice applying the matrix to this same process. On the diagram below, please label the *results* in terms of *cause and effect* as the process moves ahead.

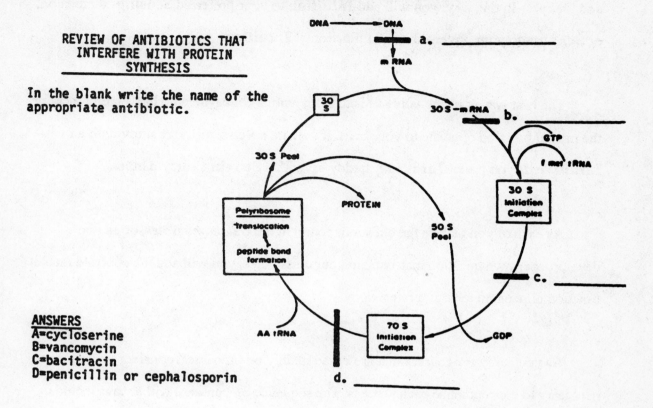

```
REVIEW OF ANTIBIOTICS THAT
   INTERFERE WITH PROTEIN
          SYNTHESIS
```

In the blank write the name of the appropriate antibiotic.

```
ANSWERS
A=cycloserine
B=vancomycin
C=bacitracin
D=penicillin or cephalosporin
```

In the space below, draw the process and label the *pivotal places* in the process, which *split* in two or more directions.

With a different colored pen, please add and label the antibiotic inhibitors.

It is natural for **Sensing (S)** types to ask "What?" of the process. **Intuitives (N)** ask "Why?" To cover all aspects of the process, ask yourself both "*What* is happening?" and "*Why?*" In this way, you will add **Intuition** to your preferred **Sensing** dimension, or **Sensing** to your preferred mental function of **Intuition**.

The best way to check yourself is to study with a colleague who has a preference for the mental function opposite to your own. If you are a **Sensing** type, study with an **Intuitive**. If you prefer **Intuition**, buddy up with a **Sensing** study partner.

As each of you tackles the questions found in the *Oklahoma Notes*, or as you develop your own question matrix from your class notes, you will add the opposite mental function dimension to your strategies.

As you study for courses that are based mainly on processes, consider the *sequence* necessary to conceptualize each process. The sequence of a process will always include:

1. the number of steps in the process
2. the requirement (cause) necessary to get from one step to the other
3. the results (effect) that occur when these requirements are activated
4. the splitting off or the merging of the process
5. the requirements that are necessary for either the branching off or the coalescence to occur.

As soon as you consider a sequence, you must begin to think like a **Sensing** type.

When you are asked questions that require you to develop a hypothesis, again you will need to look for the relationship between *cause* and *effect*. You will need to consider the *requirements* that are necessary for the expected effect to occur. You will need to ask yourself, *"What would happen if the requirements were missing?"*

Because you will be asked questions that direct you to develop hypotheses, you might as well fit your study patterns to the expectations of the exam. This will compel you to think like an **Intuitive** type.

To illustrate these principles, let's consider two questions. The first of them, question #46, is found on page 61 of the Oklahoma Notes, *Review of Physiology*. This is an example of an **Intuitive**-type question. The word "may" implies that you will need to develop a hypothesis. You will need to ask yourself *"If this, then what?"*

Let's think this through together.

46.   *Activation* of the medullary (bulbar) reticular formation **may**

    A. *desynchronize* the EEG

    B. *inhibit* myotatic reflexes

    C. *increase* respiratory rate

    D. *increase* muscle tone

    E. *increase* blood pressure

Notice that I have italicized special words in the stem and in the answer choices. They are all action words indicating a *cause* and a *result*. As you study, remember to look for this cause-effect pattern. **Intuitives (N's)** do this naturally.

O.K. By now you want the answer. It appears on page 71 of the Oklahoma Notes,

Review of Physiology. It reads: "46. Answer is B. This indicates inhibition or depression. All other events listed would occur with the activation of the pontine-mesencephalic RF."

Now for a **Sensing**-type question. Remember that this kind of question will ask you to recall details and look for relationships. Look with me at question #5 on page 170 of the Oklahoma Notes, *Review of Gross Anatomy.*

5. In the axilla,

1. the largest branch of the axillary artery *is* the subscapular artery.

2. the axillary nerve, from the posterior cord of the brachial plexus, *passes* into the quadrangular space with the posterior humeral circumflex artery of the axillary artery.

3. a nerve from C5-7 *is found* on the surface of serratus anterior.

4. the middle subscapular nerve *courses* downward to innervate teres major.

Notice that I have indicated the verbs in italics. These verbs all relate to how things *are* in the here and now, where they are located, where they start, where they go, and where they end.

These verbs reflect phenomena you can *see*. When you answer a question with your five senses, you are engaging your **Sensing (S)** mental function. Therefore, the **Sensing** types are right at home with this kind of material.

Now that you are sure of how your perceiving (**S** and **N**) mental functions work, how about the other dimension that you revealed in your questionnaire: your attitude about making decisions? What does your **Judging (J)** or **Perceiving (P)** dimension reveal?

Judging (J) and Perceiving (P)

Remember the question:

"Do you tend to prefer

A) closure and the settling of things, or

B) keeping options open so you can go with the flow?"

People who prefer closure are called **Judging (J)** types, whereas those who prefer to keep their options open in order to gather more data are called **Perceiving (P)** types.

If your answers to the questions reveal that you prefer **Judging**, you will feel uncomfortable until you have made a decision. Once the decision is made, you will relax. As a **J**, you like to plan ahead, meet deadlines, and have your "ducks all in a row." **J**'s enjoy completion, prefer organization, are deliberate, structured, and like control. Give **J**'s a deadline, and they will have the job done ahead of time. Their Christmas cards are addressed during their summer vacation.

The **Perceiving (P)** types, on the other hand, will resist decisions until the last minute. They like to live in a flexible, spontaneous way. If you are a **P**, no matter how much research you have gathered, you feel that you have insufficient data for optimal decision-making. **P** types enjoy gathering experiences, become enlivened by discoveries, and tend to go with the flow. For them, life is a journey, not a destination. **P**'s are adaptable and curious. They seek to understand life rather than control it.

Deadlines for **P**'s are timely guideposts but not mandates. Given an urgent deadline, they get the job done, but they may "pull an all-nighter" to do it, then rush to the post office to have the stamp canceled before midnight. Their Christmas cards are addressed by the last week of December. If Leonardo da Vinci were a **P**, he would still be adjusting Mona Lisa's smile.

The **P** person will feel uneasy and restless after making a decision. The **J** type, in the same situation, will feel relieved and fulfilled once decisions are out of the way.

J's and **P**'s show a difference in their attitude toward work:

Judging types feel that work comes first. Theirs is a work ethic. Work must be completed before time is allowed for rest or play. **J**'s willingly tackle preparation, maintenance, and cleanup; they accept the reality of these tasks as necessary aspects of the job. Planfully, they will schedule their work, and they will faithfully adhere to the schedule.

Perceiving types seem to have a play ethic, interspersing work and play. If the work process flows well, the more the better, especially if it's fun. But as for preparation, maintenance, and cleanup, **P**'s seem to shrug and say, "That's not too important to the task." You can see how this might affect the study habits of **Perceivers**. **P**'s *will* study, but not necessarily with any set "habits." When working, **P**'s frequently find themselves expanding their attention to areas beyond the actual tasks they set out to accomplish.

J's will tend to stay focused on the subject matter, study just enough, and then move on to the next task. **P**'s may find themselves probing endlessly into areas of interest and have difficulty moving on. **J**'s may not go deeply enough into the subject matter, and come to completion too soon. **P**'s may probe and dawdle too much, and not get to attend to all of the material.

The following illustration depicts the differences in study patterns of **J**'s and **P**'s. **J** types will look up a word in the dictionary, find it, and return to their writing, immediately applying the word. **P** types will look up a word, get interested in the next word on the page and then the next. Before they know it, the **P**'s will have read the whole page of the dictionary before returning to the identified word to put it to use. In Chapter Two • Time Management and Memory, this need for exploration that **P**'s exhibit will be addressed in depth.

There are special caveats for **Judgers** and **Perceivers** making examination decisions. Because they like to come to conclusions, **J**'s tend to make decisions about answers too quickly. If you are a **J,** to improve your test results you will need to read exam questions thoroughly before deciding on the answer. The techniques necessary for this procedure will be discussed in Chapter Seven • Test-Taking and Discrimination Skills.

Because they have difficulty coming to closure, **P**'s tend to overread questions. They look for material that is not present in the question as it is presented. For example, ask a **P** type, "Where is the floor in relation to the ceiling? Is the ceiling up, and the floor down?" **P**'s can reason that there are times when the ceiling is down and the floor is up. . . . How? "Well, at night, when the earth rotates on its axis," they will argue, "the juxtaposition will shift the room so that ceiling is down and floor is up! Not only that," they may argue, "but the ceiling of this room is part of the floor above this room, therefore, the ceiling is down from the floor above. . . ." And so on.

Additional Myers-Briggs Learning Style Dimensions

The four dimensions **S, N, J,** and **P** are not all you need to know about yourself. There are other aspects of your personality type that are revealed in the Myers-Briggs Type Indicator.

The two other mental functions--**Thinking (T)** and **Feeling (F)**--and information about the source of your energy--**Extraversion (E)** and **Introversion (I)**--will need to be considered.

Extraversion and Introversion

The terms **Extravert** and **Introvert** identify the source of your energy while you interact with the world. Where you like to focus your attention will determine whether you will classify yourself as preferring **Extraversion** or **Introversion**.

The words "extravert" and "introvert" have emotionally charged meanings in our society. An **Extravert** is not necessarily the back-slapping, pushy used-car salesman. Nor does the term **Introvert** imply a socially inept "nerd." Both **Extraverts** and **Introverts** are valuable and personable. Both **E's** and **I's** like and need people, but in different doses and at different times. Both make good friends, capable scientists, and fine physicians. Do you believe that you are an **Extravert** or an **Introvert**?

Let's find out about your preference for **Extraversion** or **Introversion**.

Based on their meaning, select your choice from word pairs that follow:

1. Outer	Inner
2. With others	Alone
3. Interaction	Concentration
4. Breadth	Depth
5. Verbal	Silent
6. Action	Introspection
7. Many relationships	Few relationships
8. Do	Reflect
9. Accessible	Remote
10. Gregarious	Intimate

If the words on the left appeal to you for their meaning, then you can probably classify yourself as preferring **Extraversion**. If those on the right resonate with your psyche, then you probably prefer **Introversion**.

E's need to *experience* the world in order to understand it. As a result, **E**'s will tend to take action. Inner-directed **I**'s like to *understand* the world fully before experiencing it, and will delay action until their understanding is complete.

Obviously, depending on circumstances, all of us need to spend time with others and time alone, using both **Extraversion** and **Introversion**. Our preferred energy source is inborn and will cause us to use one or the other more often if we are left to our own devices. See which of the descriptions on the next page, **E** or **I**, applies to you.

Extraversion (E)

In the formulation of ideas, **Extraverts** become animated by talking through ideas with others. **E**'s talk *as* they think; therefore, they tend to respond to a question immediately. Because their thinking is an externalized process, **E**'s may change their minds as they answer a question. They require sociability and are energized by talking, playing, and working with people. **Extraverts** will feel lonely and depleted when they are alone too long.

Students who are **E**'s prefer to study in the company of others. They place their desks so that they can look out the window. The door to their room is usually open. **E**'s tire rapidly if they are confined to solitary study activity.

They do well when they study in the library, where they can be energized by seeing what others are doing, but they must discipline themselves not to become distracted by their sociability needs.

Introversion (I)

Those who prefer **Introversion** attend more to their inner world. They are charged by the emotional and intellectual work that goes on privately inside their heads. **I**'s produce their creative energy by dipping into themselves. Although they can and do interact with others, it is their internal processes that excite and enliven them.

Becoming drained of energy when compelled to interact in large groups, they can become lonely in a crowd. When they are forced into a populated situation, like a party or a large group meeting, **I**'s will try to find one other person for conversation, or they will withdraw. In large groups, they will become tired and seek solitude in order to recharge their emotional batteries.

I 's think through ideas *before* they speak; therefore, when asked a question, they will require time for reflection. In answering questions, they offer the finished product of their internal work.

Rarely will you find I 's willingly studying in the company of others. They guard themselves against energy invasion and prefer to study alone. I 's are territorial about their space. When at their desks, I 's often shield their eyes behind their hands. Their doors are closed. The library is used by I 's as a resource center, not a study location.

Application of E and I in Examination Preparation

As you prepare for the practice of medicine, your education process is a time-pressured balancing act. By now you have discovered that you must learn to be proficient in managing time and you must be selective in your focus on the massive amount of material that you must master. You may have found that working alone is more time-efficient than working with others. I 's have no trouble with this.

While you prepare for National Boards, however, beware of the dangers in working alone all the time. When you work alone, you may not be able to consider all the dimensions of a subject. For complete coverage of the material, whether you are an E or an I, you will need to balance your alone time with study-partner time.

Remember, when we discussed S and N, we said that if you prefer **Sensing**, you may not add the "What would happen if . . .?" questions that come naturally to the

Intuitive. Conversely, if you prefer **Intuition**, you may not be noticing all the details that are the forte of the **Sensing** types. Therefore, to cover all of the *details* (**S**) and *concepts* (**N**), you must arrange your time to include work with a study partner who favors the complementary or opposite mental function.

To make optimal use of all of the possibilities to be derived from external and internal aspects of the study process, find a study partner who is your opposite in the "energy source" (**E** or **I**) aspect of your personality type.

If you are an **Introvert**, you will do well to find an **Extraverted** partner who will talk through the study tasks. Examination proficiency requires *externalization* of your study efforts.

If you are an **Extravert**, you will need the **Introvert** to help you *internalize* and summarize the finished products of your study process. For maximum complementarity of talents, the ideal study-partner combination is **Introverted Intuitive** with **Extraverted Sensor**, or **Extraverted Intuitive** with **Introverted Sensor**.

Thinking and Feeling

Now let us address the other two mental functions, **Thinking** (**T**) and **Feeling** (**F**). Consider the meanings of the words on the next page.

Indicate your preference for one word of each pair as they appear on the left and right:

1. Objective	Subjective
2. Head	Heart
3. Justice	Harmony
4. Principles	Values
5. Criticize	Appreciate
6. Analyze	Empathize
7. Laws	Extenuating circumstances
8. Precision	Persuasion
9. Standards	Good or bad
10. Impersonal	Personal

If more of the words in the left column appeal to you, you probably prefer **Thinking.** If those on the right strike your fancy, then **Feeling** is the mental function you prefer.

The **T** and **F** functions refer to the mental process you employ when you make decisions. If you make decisions impersonally and tend to be *objective* when you evaluate matters, you are most likely a **T** type. If, on the other hand, you make choices based on your personal values and tend to be more *subjective*, you probably can classify yourself as an **F** type.

To illustrate the use of **Thinking** and **Feeling** in an everyday interaction, I will let you in on a vignette that might take place in my personal life: If I were to ask my husband, an engineer who prefers **Thinking**, "How do I look?" he would inspect me and say,

"Your hair is straggling in the back. Fix it." (Objectively true.) He cares about me, and because he cares, he will use his ability to criticize and analyze while making this evaluation of my appearance.

In the unlikely event that he would ask me the same question, I, being a **Feeling**-type psychotherapist, would say, "You look terrific! I'm sure that you will make a great impression on your client." (Subjectively supportive.) I care about him, too, and because I care, I will use my ability to be affirming and reassuring.

Thinkers are fair, but they do not necessarily trouble themselves about people's feelings when they are being fair. **Feelers** value affiliation and harmony, so they will tend to temper their objectivity with subjective concern for the emotional reactions of others.

Both ways of selecting alternatives when evaluating what to do or not to do--**T** and **F**--are necessary and useful. When we take action, all of us use both objectivity and subjectivity. But as with the mental functions **S** and **N**, we *prefer* one or the other. Therefore, we tend to use our preferred mental function more than we use our less-developed mental function. Misunderstandings between **Thinkers** and **Feelers** can be avoided if the differences in the points of view are understood.

In clinical decision-making, and in communicating with patients, patients' families, and your own families, **Thinking** and **Feeling** dimensions are more important than they are in your preclinical study/test venue. For that reason, we will not delve into the application of the **T** and **F** dimensions at this time.

DETERMINING YOUR TYPE

You have now completed the initial process of identifying some aspects of your preferred Learning Style. You have disclosed the mental functions you use while perceiving information and making decisions about information. You have determined your energy source, and your attitude toward coming to closure on decisions.

Your personal choices have revealed your personality type, which can be represented by a four-letter shorthand symbol. Let's construct that symbol by proceeding step by step.

1. Use the letter **E** If you prefer to get your energy from the *external* world. Use **I** if your energy is derived *internally*. Circle one or the other.   **E**   or   **I**

2. Now your preferred mental functions **S** for *details* or **N** for *concepts*. Which one have you identified as your preference? Circle one or the other.   **S**   or   **N**
Combine this letter with the previous one.
By now you have chosen **ES** or **IS, EN** or **IN.**

3. If you prefer the *objective* method of making decisions, use **T**. If you tend to be *subjective*, choose **F**. Circle one.   **T**   or   **F**
Add the **T** or **F** to get: **EST** or **ESF; ENT** or **ENF; IST** or **ISF; INT** or **INF.**

4. Now for the final dimension, your attitude toward making decisions: **J** indicates a preference for coming to *closure,* and **P** signifies a preference for keeping options *open*. Add that letter, too.   **J**   or   **P**

You have identified yourself as one of the following 16 types:

ESTJ or **ESTP**; **ESFJ** or **ESFP**; **ENTJ** or **ENTP**; **ENFJ** or **ENFP**;

ISTJ or **ISTP**; **ISFT** or **ISFP**; **INFJ** or **INFP**; **INTJ** or **INTP**.

Which one are you? Please write your selection in the space below.

My four-letter type is: _____

You will refer to this four-letter code when you apply your Learning Style to the chapters that follow.

If you feel that you came out with a tie score, move your score in the direction of **I**, **N**, **F**, and **P**. Because there are cultural pulls in the direction of **E**, **S**, **T**, and **J**, the research in psychological type tells us that we should break any tie by adding a point to the direction that is not culturally weighted (Myers and McCaulley, 1985).

Because they have not yet developed a strong preference for either polarity, people whose scores are tied report that they often feel ambivalent and unsettled when they must apply the dimensions in which they have tie scores.

For instance, if your score is tied on **Judging** and **Perceiving**, when you make decisions you may feel that you have decided too quickly, while simultaneously feeling as though you have taken too long to come to conclusions. As you develop one or the other dimension, you will gain skill and confidence in that area.

PERCEPTUAL PREFERENCE

In addition to the psychological type information about your energy source (**E** or **I**), your mental functions (**S** or **N**, **T** or **F**), and your attitude toward making decisions (**J** or **P**), which constitute your four-letter type identification, let's attend to other important dimensions of your learning style. How do your perceptual preferences affect your learning?

When you are confronted with new ideas, what aspects of your sensory or motor system do you use to attend to information and make sense of what you've learned? Your perceptual preference or a combination of sensory categories of perception and communication will determine what you tend to observe (Spitz, 1965).

Are you a **Visual, Aural/Oral, Kinetic, Gustatory**, or **Tactile** learner? Hobbies, pastimes, and interests can be reliable indicators of which sense you tend to enjoy using. When you are learning new information, you will tend to use that preferred sense to help you take in new data. Which sense do you think you prefer?

Write your guess: _____

Perhaps you can't decide. You like the visual arts, enjoy the sounds of music, and tend to like to exercise and dance. Psychological studies inform us that engaging the full use of all of your sensory possibilities will maximize learning (Ausabel, 1960; Dellarosa and Bourne, 1985; Galbraith and James, 1986).

In my experience counseling medical students, once students identify the methods they use naturally, and begin to use these methods systematically and with purpose, they learn more quickly and retain the information longer (Shain and Kelliher, 1988).

You may be unaware of using any particular sense other than your analytic capacities. For purposes of helping you to appreciate and use your preferred sense to your full educational advantage, we will over simplify a complex phenomenon of educational psychology--perceptual preference--by using the following examples.

Visual

What are your interests and pastimes? Do your interests pull you toward visual pursuits? Do you have a hobby that uses your talent and ability to see? Do you like art, architecture, fashion, and photography?

In your interactions with others, do you tend to visualize what they are saying? When someone asks you a question, do you indicate your understanding by saying, "I see"? When you ask a passerby for street directions, do you prefer to have directions pointed out on a map so you can *see* them, rather than receive them verbally?

If you are such an individual, when you try to recall what you have studied you will close your eyes and see the colors and positions of the printed words on the page. You will label your notes with different colors for maximum recall.

Because of your need to *see,* for maximum comprehension and recall, you need to write and rewrite your notes when you memorize. If this sounds like you, then call yourself **Visual**.

Aural/Oral

Think about whether your hobbies and methods of relaxation engage your hearing. Do you find yourself humming when you relax? If you enjoy music and are soothed by the refrains of wind chimes, if conversational voice tones and alliterations remain in your head, if you can imitate accents and musical pitches, if the sounds of the world intrigue you, you enjoy using your hearing/saying, aural/oral capacity to experience the world.

Because of your well-developed aural/oral acuity, you "tune in" to yourself and others. When you ask for street directions, you have no trouble remembering the spoken word, especially if you *hear* yourself repeat the directions.

When someone tells you about an idea he has, or a feeling he's experiencing, you will affirm your understanding by saying, "I hear you."

Chances are that you also use your hearing to learn. When you study, you find yourself reciting aloud as you memorize. You may vary your speaking pitch, or even sing to emphasize important areas.

As you read through your study material, you tend to remember the intonation of the teacher's voice as you recall the lecture. Articulated verbalizations, both yours and other folks, is a necessary component of your comprehension skills and memorization techniques.

Is this you? If so, call yourself **Aural/Oral**.

Kinetic

Do you take pleasure in the movements of the world? Do you enjoy dancing, aerobic exercise, swimming? Do the rhythms of landscapes stay with you? In your physical self-expression, are you able to let your mind take second place to your body's activity? Does sitting for long periods make you uncomfortable unless you can stretch or shift your position?

When you are traveling, you might not want to ask others for street directions, preferring instead to experience the movement of the journey. Should you become hopelessly lost and allow yourself to ask for directions, you may notice that your hand and body motions mimic the course of the directives you receive. As you hear the words "turn right," your arms and head may tend to move in that direction.

You may gesture when you speak. When someone gives you information or confides in you, you may affirm your understanding by some form of body motion like nodding or slapping your side. To affirm your understanding of what is being told to you, you may say, "I follow you." When you feel something deeply, you may need to become physically active to let off steam. Or, if you are pressed to verbalize a reaction, you might say,"I feel moved."

If these are your tendencies, you need to pace, move, or be on your feet when you study. You often tap your pencil on the page while you think. As you remember a lecture, you recall the gestures of your professor. In order to comprehend information, you need to "place it" physically within a context.

You do well using gross motor activity when you memorize. Rather than restrict yourself to notebook paper, you achieve better study results when you write on a large surface like a blackboard. You may snap your fingers and swing your arms when you recall the steps of a process. You use your hands to shape structures in the air.

Is this an accurate description of you? Then call yourself **Kinetic.**

Gustatory

You may find that the tastes you experience are important to you. Your hobbies include restaurant-going, cooking, eating, spice and perfume collecting. You "sniff out" or "sink your teeth into" information. When someone tells you a story you can't fathom, you may use an expression like "Do you expect me to swallow that?"

Gustatory people tend to chew or eat while they study. If you are gustatory, you may find yourself making associations to food as you incorporate new knowledge with the old. One student told her study-group classmates that the only way she could memorize the steps of any process--like those of the Krebs cycle--was to recite them while she turned a spoon in mixing cake batter. You, like this student, may see collections of facts as ingredients. You may need to make associations to tastes and smells as you study.

Some gustatory students have said that they will chew different-flavored chewing gums as they ruminate difficult subject areas. They cannot master anatomy without spearmint gum, or physiology without Juicy Fruit. When memorizing the parts of a structure, gustatory types may use peanuts, Cheerios, raisins, or any small chewable to incorporate the individual parcels of a large knowledge area. Ten parts? Ten raisins!

If you are a gustatory type, when you acknowledge your understanding of an idea or a concept, you will talk about "digesting" the information. When you are asked to recall memorized material, you may refer to this process as "regurgitation." If this sounds like you, call yourself **Gustatory**.

Tactile

Your hobbies include activities that enable you to touch, fondle, and mold things in your hands. Sculpting, wood carving, kneading, and sewing may be your method of relaxation. You notice surfaces and textural differences. Smooth, rough, or multitextured fabrics, cool and hard surfaces, cushy pillows capture your attention.

When you study anatomy, you will remember best if you personally have felt the structures between your fingers. In courses requiring you to visualize abstractions, you do well if you construct models that you can touch to represent a process.

During study and test-taking sessions, the clothing you wear and the furniture supporting you must be texturally friendly for you to do your best. Your writing instruments must feel comfortable in your hand.

Does this sound like you? Then call yourself **Tactile**.

SUMMARY

People experience the world in many ways. We learn through our minds, our senses, and our bodies. Now that you have identified your learning style, you can appreciate and apply your preferred methods of experiencing the world to your study and test-taking strategies.

Most of us combine activities as we learn. To derive energy, we externalize and internalize (**E** and **I**). We attend to details and concepts (**S** and **N**). We are objective and subjective (**T** and **F**). We come to closure and try to leave options open (**J** and **P**). We see, say, hear, pace, take hold, and munch as we learn.

By now you know your multifaceted Learning Style. You know if you are a **Visual ISTP**, an **Aural/Oral ESTJ**, a **Tactile ENFP**, a **Gustatory INTJ**, or ONE of the OTHER possible combinations of mind/body learning. Please write your learning style type below.

Learning Style: _____.

You will facilitate your progress and prevent study burnout if you consciously use this information by integrating your playful, relaxed self in your serious, performance-based settings.

If your learning style is not fully developed, or if you still aren't sure of how to classify your learning style, perhaps you have been trying to emulate the techniques of your family or of successful colleagues. These techniques may not fit your innate learning style. Be yourself.

All of your talents and limitations make you valuable and unique. Give yourself permission to appreciate what *you* do while you study and while you retrieve information. The more *active* you are as you practice your study, recall, and test-taking techniques, the more successful you will be (Kiewra, et al., 1991; McKeachie, 1990;).

Using all of your favorite sensual, intellectual, and energy-producing talents as you study will provide you with success and pleasure during the many phases of your lifelong learning journey. The following chapters will guide you through this process.

References

Ausabel, D.P. (1960) The use of advance organizers in the learning and retention of meaningful verbal material. *Journal of Educational Psychology*, 51, pp 267-272

Dellarosa, D. and Bourne, L.E. (1985) Surface form and spacing effect. *Memory and Cognition*, 13, pp 529-537

Fratzka, B. J. (1989) A study of the relationship between preferred learning style and personality type among traditional age college students and adult learners. *Dissertation Abstracts International* 49 (12-A, Pt. 1) p 3587

Galbraith, M. and James, W. B. (1986) Techniques for assessing perceptual learning style. *Activities, Adaptation and Aging* 8 (2) pp 29-38

Jung, C. (1923) *Psychological Types* New York: Harcourt Brace

Kiewra, K. A., Mayer, R. E., Christensen, M., Kim, S., and Risch, N. (1991) Effects of repetition on recall and notetaking; strategies for learning from lectures, *Journal of Educational Psychology* Vol 83 No. (1) pp 120-123

Leon, R. and Martinez, F. (1989) Recent Developments in Medical Education At The Universidad Autonoma De Guadalajara School Of Medicine. Wash., D.C. Innovations in Medical Education, American Association of Medical Colleges

McKeachie, W. J. (1990) Research on college teaching: The historical background. *Journal of Educational Psychology* 82 (2) pp 189-200

Myers, I. B. and McCaulley, M. H. (1985) *Manual: A Guide to the Development and Use of the Myers-Briggs Type Indicator.* Palo Alto, CA: Consulting Psychologists Press

Provost, J. A. and Anchors, S. (1987) *Applications of the Myers-Briggs Type Indicator in Higher Education.* Palo Alto, CA: Consulting Psychologists Press

Shain, D. D. and Kelliher, G. J. (1988) A study skills workshop as an integral part of orientation to medical school: The establishment of self-directed learning. *Proceedings of the Twenty-Seventh Annual Conference Research in Medical Education* Chicago, Illinois. Assoc. of Amer. Medical Colleges pp 91-96

Spitz, R. A. (1965) *The First Year of Life: A Psychological Study of Normal and Deviant Development of Object Relations.* New York: International Universities Press

Suggested Readings

Dunn, R. and Griggs, S. (1990) Research on learning style characteristics of selected racial and ethnic groups. *Journal of Reading, Writing and learning Disabilities* 6 (3) pp 261-280

Hyde, R. M. (1987) *Microbiology and Immunology: Oklahoma Notes.* New York: Springer-Verlag

Keirsey, D. and Bates, M. (1984) *Please Understand Me: Character and Temperament Types.* Del Mar, CA: Prometheus Nemisis Book Company

Lyman, H. B. (1986) *Test Scores and What They Mean* Englewood Cliffs, NJ: Prentice-Hall

McCaulley, M. H. (1987) *Developing Critical Thinking and Problem-Solving Abilities: New Directions for Teaching and Learning,* San Francisco: Jossey-Bass

Myers, I. B. and Briggs, K. C. (1976, 1988) *Myers Briggs Type Indicator,* Palo Alto, CA: Consulting Psychologists Press, Inc.

Myers, I. B. (1980) *Gifts Differing* .Palo Alto, CA: Consulting Psychologists Press

Person, R. J. and Theis, R. (1989) *Physiology : Oklahoma Notes.* New York: Springer-Verlag

Piaget, J. (1950) *The Psychology of Intelligence.* M. Piercy and D.E. Berlyne, Trans. London: Keigan Paul, Trench, and Trubner

Shain, D. D. (1989) Self-directed learning and collegial interaction through the use of the Myers-Briggs Type Indicator in medical education. In *Proceedings APT VIII Biennial International Conference, Boulder CO Frontiers of Psychological Type* Gainsville, FL Association for Psychological Type pp 101-104

Stice, J. E. (1987) *Developing Critical Thinking and Problem-Solving Abilities* San Franciso: Jossey-Bass Inc

Wessells, M. G. (1982) *Cognitive Psychology.* New York: Harper and Row

CHAPTER TWO • TIME MANAGEMENT AND MEMORY

Professional success requires skillful time management and a good memory. As a physician, you will need to organize your schedule to handle all you want to do: see patients, keep current with journals and medical research, socialize with family and friends, exercise, keep healthy, and know your craft while trying to remain human. How will you accomplish all this? You start now as a physician-in-training.

In medical school, there are too many facts to remember and too little time to analyze and synthesize the ever-growing information explosion. Time, timing, and memory work together. Once you take charge and master time-management techniques, you will learn more and retain information longer. "The doctor must develop a personal systematic approach to science, to medicine, and the best use of time. Since all three are interrelated and mastery is influenced by the capacities of the individual and the nature of the practice, each physician must work out a personal plan" (Houle, 1984).

Purpose

This chapter will enable you to use a conscious system of time-conserving study steps. The system is designed to increase your short-term and long-term memory, ensuring success in course work and the National Boards. You will learn to set realistic short-term goals and to use specific strategies of scheduling and long-term planning.

On completion of this chapter, you will understand and apply seven basic principles:

1. time management
2. the memory curve
3. schedule construction
4. selecting study tasks

5. using your learning style
6. time accountability
7. study tricks and treats.

TIME MANAGEMENT

In the lifelong learning process necessary for the practice of medicine, you must be time-efficient. As a medical student, you begin this process by finding ways to save time while you commit material to short-term memory for daily course work and long-term memory for the National Board Examinations. Like a long-distance runner, you need to pace yourself as you control each step along the path leading to the finish line--the achievement of your M.D. degree and, ultimately, the responsible practice of medicine (Wolf et al., 1980).

Unlike undergraduate school, where the work load allowed you to use time elastically, in medical school there is simply too much material to cover in the time allowed. As an undergraduate, you had about two weeks to cover what you are expected to master in one day of medical school (Canaday and Lancaster, 1985).

Bright undergraduates have plenty of time to party and play, putting on the study steam by pulling all-nighters just before an exam. In medical school, however, mental meandering followed by all-night study sessions will not provide you with the time you need to master all the work. Nor will cram sessions result in the long-term memory necessary for National Boards.

As a physician-in-training, don't expect to be whipped into action by teacher-determined *external* control. The only one who will really care if you study will be you. Unless you take *internal* control of your time, you will be forever in a management-by-crisis time frenzy. Management by crisis is the modus operandi for many **Intuitive** and **Perceiving** types. For each hour of class time, you need to spend two hours of self-directed study.

Self-monitored, planned study steps will save you time, increase your long-term memory, and improve your examination scores. Are you ready to try this new and efficient time-management method? Let's begin by demonstrating some useful principles of the psychology of learning--the *memory curve*. Mastering the memory curve means applying specific time-conserving techniques.

THE MEMORY CURVE

The memory curve is an imaginary line illustrating the process of remembering and forgetting. It climbs with study exposure, drops with neglect, and moves up again with relearning. Depending on the timing and frequency of specific memory reinforcers, this line can form a constant upward curve, or it can be as erratic and scary as a rollercoaster ride.

Because rollercoasters are inefficient modes of memory transportation, your goal is to create an ever-upward *optimal* memory curve, a steadily rising slant achieved through well-timed, planned, and disciplined reinforcement of mastered material. Optimal memory curve techniques demand that you pay attention to the timing of reinforcers and to the specific methods you use to secure short-term and long-term memory.

Achieving the optimal memory curve takes practice. Not only does practice make perfect, but time of practice is key. To illustrate the creation of an optimal memory curve, let's use two common examples:

1. learning to play a musical instrument

2. learning to speak a foreign language.

Example #1: Music

You play a passage of music on your instrument. At your lesson, the teacher corrects your fingering or your phrasing. In order to remember the revision, you must reinforce your new learning by *immediately* replaying the passage correctly at least three times. It will also help your memory if you tap your foot or sing along as you reinforce the learning.

Example #2: Foreign Language

You say a sentence. Your grammar is incorrect. Someone corrects you. In order to recall the correct usage, you must *immediately* repeat the sentence properly, saying it at least three times. You can pace or tap your finger while you repeat the sentence. You might want to use the sentence in a different paragraph. If you are a visual learner, you will find that writing the sentence in a notebook will lock it in your memory.

In both examples, the *immediacy, frequency,* and *variety* of reinforcers--hearing, doing, saying, seeing, and moving- can make the difference between short-term learning or forgetting. So, for example, if you are a **Visual Intuitive** type of learner, first reinforce your learning through visualized concepts, then deepen your learning by adding a repetition of details through your less developed **Aural/Oral Sensing** dimensions. Reinforce and expand your learning-style dimensions immediately after you learn something new.

To achieve long-term memory, you will want to break large tasks down into smaller ones. Reinforce over a long period of time. Set deadlines and priorities. Use waiting time efficiently. Avoid interruptions and guard against procrastination. Increase efficiency by combining tasks, and most important--adhere to a routine of memory reinforcement.

This routine includes specific tasks you need to do before class, during class, and after class each day. By following a routine, you will use less time to remember large amounts of material. You want to create an optimal memory curve. To establish it, you will need to know and apply the proper order of activities during the learning process. Students who do not follow this order of activities have difficulty maintaining academic competence.

Let's look at the dysfunctional memory curve of a student in trouble. Notice how this chart has no specific study statements, and the curve fluctuates up and down rather than moving in an upward direction.

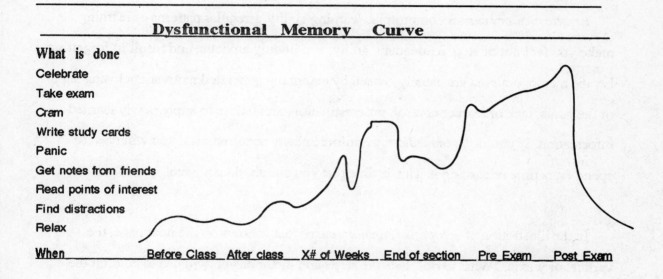

Dysfunctional Memory Curve

What is done
Celebrate
Take exam
Cram
Write study cards
Panic
Get notes from friends
Read points of interest
Find distractions
Relax

When   Before Class After class X# of Weeks End of section Pre Exam Post Exam

In my years as a medical education counselor, I have found, as have other medical educators, that students in academic difficulty have not learned how to manage time or material (Wolf et al., 1980). In counseling sessions with students in trouble, I discovered that they had a number of blocks to learning. Most of them simply had no system of study; others allowed themselves to become distracted by getting overinvolved with outside interests such as jobs, family matters, and extracurricular activities. Only about 10 percent had unresolved psychological conflicts interfering with their progress.

48

Those few students who needed psychotherapy and sought help showed marked improvement (Alpert and Haber, 1960). About 85 percent improved greatly when they took action and developed a systematic study regimen. They developed organized habits adhering to a planned and timely course of study reinforcement. Once they set short-term and long-term goals, limited their socializing, and took responsibility for their own behavior, they succeeded. Only about 5 percent of students in academic difficulty get into trouble because they don't have the intelligence or background to get through medical school (Montecinos and Jackson, 1987).

Erratic memory curves compromise learning ability. Irregular patterns of learning make you feel out of step, inadequate, guilty, and unduly anxious, and result in forgetting. Erratic memory curves are usually caused by externally generated motivation, losing sight of the goals, lack of learner control, procrastination, and failure to apply newly learned information. If you don't *immediately* reinforce newly acquired data, you will need to spend extra time relearning it. This is time that you simply do not have!

In the illustration of an *optimal memory curve* that follows on the next page, the vertical or y axis, "What to do," lists the steps and methods you will use to commit the material to memory.

The horizontal or x axis, "When to do it," represents specific points in time and plots the most advantageous time for reinforcing new information. After you see the steps presented in the memory curve diagram, we will go through the steps systematically.

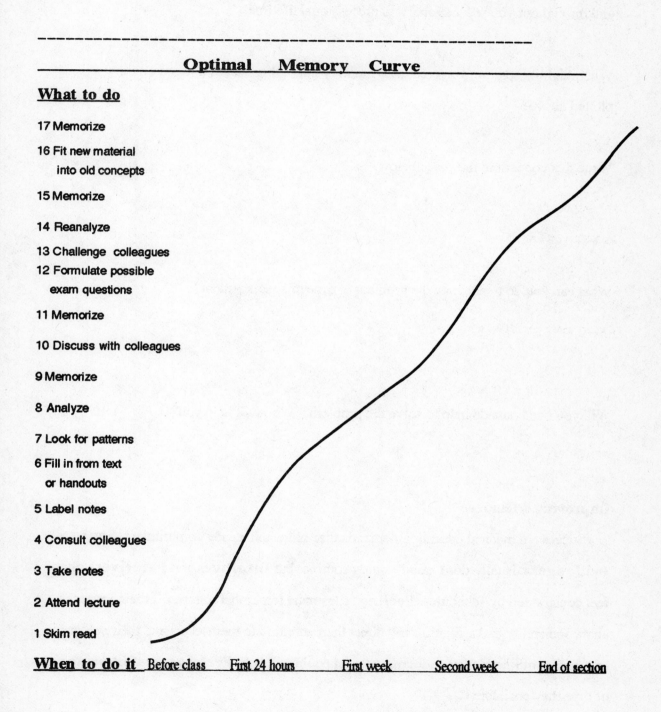

Optimal   Memory   Curve

What to do

17 Memorize

16 Fit new material
   into old concepts

15 Memorize

14 Reanalyze

13 Challenge colleagues

12 Formulate possible
   exam questions

11 Memorize

10 Discuss with colleagues

9 Memorize

8 Analyze

7 Look for patterns

6 Fill in from text
   or handouts

5 Label notes

4 Consult colleagues

3 Take notes

2 Attend lecture

1 Skim read

When to do it Before class   First 24 hours   First week   Second week   End of section

Steps 1-6, exposure and analysis, should take place within the first 24 hours of meeting new material. Activities 7-13, memorization and synthesis, occur within the first week. Items 14-17, consolidation, will take place within the first month of information exposure and throughout your educational and professional lifetime.

What might keep you from creating a memory curve that moves upward on the y axis as plotted above?

Write that concern in the space below:

What can you do to alleviate the problem of time mismanagement?

Will you need outside help to solve the problem? Who will help you?

Improving Memory

Success in medical education demands discipline and steady commitment. **Sensors** and **Judgers** usually don't mind a study routine, but **Intuitives** and **Perceivers** often feel constrained by schedules. **Feeling** types must remember to turn off their concerns about sociability and affiliation and direct their attention to themselves and their solitary acquisition of knowledge. Adhering to a schedule will help **Feelers** to control the amount of time they socialize.

Specific Study Strategies

In learning new material, you will need to proceed with the following study steps within the first 24 hours of your initial exposure to the material.

(1) *Skim read*

Prepare for class and anticipate findings through rapid reading. Before going to class or to a board review session, quickly skim read the chapter or material that pertains to the class or review session. While swiftly flipping each page, attend to the special type, such as boldface or italicized print. Slow down to read charts, diagrams, and graphs. Read the introduction, table of contents, and summary statements. Notice if there are relationships in the material. Pay attention to compare/contrast data. Depending on the complexity of the chapter, 60-100 pages can be skim read in about 20 minutes.

In order to prevent note-taking slowdown, develop a glossary of unfamiliar terms. Scan the pages and the table of contents for words or concepts that are unfamiliar, and say them aloud. Use a medical dictionary if you feel particularly uneasy about the unfamiliar terms. In selecting a medical dictionary, you might want to look over several choices before you buy one. In my work applying learning style to study skills, **Sensors** seem to prefer Dorland and **Intuitives** like Stedman (Shain and Kelliher, 1988).

(2) *Attend lecture*

With skim reading as your map, navigate the lecture territory by going to class prepared to listen and to take notes as fast as you can. In the lecture, you will discover areas that are important to memorize and areas that can be whizzed through quickly at your second reading.

Sit in a well-lighted place so that you will not be distracted by active doorways or by colleagues' conversation. Position yourself in the front of the room so you will not be able to drift off and fall asleep.

(3) *Take notes*

One of the main goals of note-taking is to create your own text. Because the most advantageous study period is within 24 hours of exposure to new material, a personal textbook is one of the best ways to reinforce immediately what you are learning. Nothing can replace a good set of notes.

Use a fast-moving writing instrument and capture as much of the lecture as possible. Use only one side of the page so that you have space to fill in additional information on the opposite, facing page. Leave two-inch margins. Margins invite you to apply labels when you are organizing your notes at home. In Chapter Three • Taking Notes, additional techniques of note-taking and labeling are discussed.

(4) *Consult colleagues*

Immediately after class, talk with your colleagues. Go over the concepts you understand, and ask your colleagues if they can clarify points that were mystifying to you. Discussions go well with lunch or walking to and from class, while exercising, or while socializing. On the page facing your own lecture notes, write the ideas you have acquired from colleagues in a different colored ink. By distinguishing others' notes from your own, you will be able to see those areas that were unclear to you when you first met the material. These will be the areas that will need extra attention.

Remember that the best way to learn is to teach. Teach your colleagues what you know. Teaching forces you to clarify what you know and to acknowledge what you don't know. As a resident, you will be teaching as you learn. As a physician, you will spend most of your time educating your patients.

(5) *Label notes*

Labels written along the margin in contrasting colors and with a different style of writing will act as visual memory pegs. Organize details by using such identifying words as: *Structure, Function, Mechanism of Action, Mechanism, Steps of a Process, Requirements, Results, Cause-Effect, Compare/Contrast.* Use different colors for your labels--one color for *Structure,* another for *Function,* and a third for *Mechanism of Action,* etc. Color-keyed organization gives you the opportunity to visualize as you memorize efficiently.

(6) *Fill in from text or handouts*

Amplify your classroom notes. Use the space you have provided on the blank page facing your notes to deepen your understanding and widen your knowledge base. Add notes from textbooks, from handouts, and from the information you got through discussions with colleagues. Again--to improve your memory--use contrasting colors when adding new information to your original notes.

(7) *Look for patterns*

In physical objects courses, such as anatomy, notice relationships of structures to one another. Notice how structures with similar shapes perform similar functions. Observe how structure, function, and mechanism of action interact. Observe the sizes, shapes, textures, and physical and chemical linkage of structures. Where do they anastomose? Where do they bifurcate? Arrange structures in order from outside in and inside out.

In process courses, such as biochemistry, develop an information matrix containing:

• steps of the process

• requirements for the process to move forward

• results in terms of cause-effect

• reactions to too much or too little of the required component in the process

• points at which the process changes direction--where it splits or where it joins with

   another process.

(8) *Analyze*

What does all the information mean? Make it make sense by asking yourself questions about the relationship of the subjects to one another. How does anatomy, physiology, and biochemistry fit together? How might these phenomena relate to clinical implications? For a full explication of this process, see Chapter Five • Preparing For National Board Examinations.

(9) *Memorize*

Keep the memory methods in the music and foreign language examples in mind. Hearing, saying, seeing, and applying items at least three times is the bare minimum you will need to commit material to short-term memory. Successful memorization requires more than the simple intent to remember. In order to memorize successfully, you must create activities that involve all your creative capacities.

• Use all your senses

• Reread

• Rewrite

• Make compare/contrast cell charts and flow charts

• Compile flash cards

• Create mnemonics

Condensing techniques are useful tools to facilitate memorization. Carry charts and cards to be used while you wait in line at the supermarket, while you're stuck in traffic, or whenever anxiety clutches at your gut.

A word of caution: Do not spend so much time making your memory apparatus that you do not leave enough time for drilling yourself and memorizing the material you have organized on the charts or cards. Outrageous or funny mnemonics are hard to forget. But again, beware: Don't get so enamored of the mnemonics that you forget what you were attempting to memorize.

(10) *Discuss with colleagues*

Ask your friends and colleagues to review material with you. Pose to them the exam questions you constructed and ask them to quiz you. If you are an **Intuitive** student, find a **Sensor** and vice versa. If you are an **Extravert**, find an **Introvert**. In that way the two of you use thinking aloud and silent introspection to cover both the details and the concepts. You will find that memorization goes more quickly when you feel the comfort of consensus.

(11) *Memorize some more*

Use corrected charts and amplified understanding to reinforce your memorization.

(12) *Formulate possible examination questions*

All questions are derived from labels. Because simple recall questions are rarely used, create complex questions in which two labels are used together. In physical objects courses, put together the relationships of structure, function, mechanism of action, e.g., if structure changes, what happens to function? In process courses such as biochemistry or physiology, ask yourself what would happen if there was an increase or decrease in the amount of flow or a change in any aspect of the requirements necessary for the process to move forward. Ask--What will impede the process? What will hasten it? What other processes does this process depend on? For example, how does the Krebs cycle relate to glycolysis? How does the cardiac system depend on the proper workings of the renal system?

(13) *Challenge colleagues*

Review your notes and charts with opposite-type colleagues. Are you on the right track? Was your understanding the same as your colleagues' understanding? If not, why not? Pose sample exam questions to opposite-type colleagues to see if you omitted anything. Engage in scientific discourse. If colleagues' ideas differ from yours, ask them to prove their points. Be certain that you have not omitted anything.

(14) *Reanalyze*

To be certain that you have considered all the information and the relationships of one system to another, and to integrate new with known material, reanalyze the data. Use your new insights to see how the new material fits together with the old. What does the new material explain? What might be unexplained? What do you understand about the significance of the basic science material vis a vis clinical implications?

(15) *Memorize again*

Remember that memorizing each time you have added depth to your understanding sets the data in long-term memory.

(16) *Fit new material into old concepts*

To be sure that new material fits into those facts and concepts that you already know, consider various relationships and the causes and effects of changes in each system. To achieve the full picture of the knowledge you have gained, synthesize your learning. How does biochemistry impact on the physiologic aspects of the material you are studying? Anatomy and physiology?

Create questions that combine several subjects. Chapter Five • Preparing for National Board Examinations will teach you how to create a multisubject question matrix.

(17) *Memorize for long-term memory*

Reinforce the material each day. Vary the methods by which you see, do, say, analyze, and synthesize the material. Be active! If you practice the material every day during the first week of exposure, and if you use all your senses and a variety of modes of reinforcement, you will be able to cut down on study time later in the study process. Remember that more time spent early in the learning process equals less time for memory brush-ups and integration of material before exams.

You can immunize yourself against forgetting if you reinforce early in the learning process and keep intermittent reinforcing going throughout your two-year course of basic science study. At the end of each week, review the material you have learned that week and the one before. Educational psychology research shows that people retain information for decades as opposed to mere months when they learn and reinforce the material over a longer period of time, building on and reviewing the material as they go along (Adler, 1991).

If you are an auditory learner, be sure to add music to your study environment. Psychology research reveals that music and rhythmic sounds facilitate learning and the retention of verbal material over time. The background music associated with the original memorization of data can act as a cue to remembering difficult material (Bellezza, 1981; Bower and Bolton, 1969; Sims, 1980).

SCHEDULE CONSTRUCTION

To make the most efficient use of time, follow the steps outlined in the optimal memory curve. Create your personal optimal memory curve, developing a schedule based on what you know about yourself. When, and under what conditions, are you most energetic and efficient? In preparation for schedule construction, please answer the following six questions:

1. At what time of the day or night are you most alert?

2. How much sleep do you need?

3. Do you need large blocks of uninterrupted time when you work?

4. Do you find that after one and a half hours of study, you must take a break?

5. How long must the break be, and what do you like to do with the break time?

6. When do you need to study alone? When with others?

In the chart below, please note the time and the range of your energy level.

	High Energy	Moderate Energy	Low Energy

Early morning _____

Morning _____

Early afternoon _____

Late afternoon _____

Evening _____

Night_____

Late night _____

Middle of night _____

Other_____

Develop your personal schedule so that you can create a realistic study plan based on:
• the times of day in which your energy level is high and low
• your preference for large blocks of study time or hourly increments
• the activities you need to seek when you take a break
• your need for time alone and time with others.

By taking advantage of the natural ebb and flow of your energy, you will be able to use time efficiently. Tackle your most difficult study tasks when your energy is highest. Work on your favorite subjects when your energy is waning. Try not to fight your circadian rhythms, or you will waste time.

SELECTING STUDY TASKS

Narrow Your Focus

You will do well to tackle a manageable amount of material. Try to avoid global statements like: "I need to study anatomy." The use of the word "anatomy" creates a statement that is too broad. Instead, select for study a defined section of the body. Let's use, for example, the brachial plexus. Tell yourself that you will devote a specific block of time to mastering your study of *only* the nerve supply and blood supply of that region. Or resolve to study x number of pages in a subject. Stay with one topic for an hour or an hour and a half.

Work with Related Material

Once you have completed the manageable subject segment, or the realistic number of pages you have designated, intersperse this topic with a related one. If you can see connections, make the connections. If you can't, and you hit a study barrier, use your medical dictionary to spur your understanding before leaving the study section.

When you feel bogged down and want to escape a section, intersperse subjects you find difficult with others that are comfortable, familiar, and somehow related. So if you become snagged in studying a section in a process course (e.g., biochemistry), take a break and tackle a physical object course (e.g., anatomy). Be sure your selection will amplify your understanding of the troublesome area. Once you have completed this, take a break and change to a completely unrelated subject.

USING YOUR LEARNING STYLE

Control your learning environment and make it pleasant. Surround yourself with music if you are **Aural/Oral**; with warm colors and pleasing views if you are **Visual**; with satisfying tastes if you are **Gustatory**, if you are **Extraverted** seek open space; if you are **Introverted,** a secluded study setting. When you pay attention to your needs for pleasure, you will not need to escape the study location and you will save time.

Vary Sensory Use

Vary your study techniques as well as the content of your studies. Use variety in each sensory possibility.

If you are a **Visual** learner, vary colors and shapes when marking the material. Intersperse printed words with spatial models or sketches. Use both printing and cursive writing when making note cards or rewriting your notes, and vary the slant of your handwriting.

If you are **Kinetic,** pay attention to your body's needs for motion. Vary your seating, standing, and pacing position, and change study locations. Use your large muscles in gross motor activity. You can jog and stretch while you recite your material. When seated, switch chairs. Wave your arms, teaching the material to the air. Punctuate section endings with a transitional activity that includes a full range of body motion.

In addition to using 9" x 12" paper, use a chalkboard or sheets of paper the size of a newspaper page. On these larger areas, write with chalk or Magic Markers. **Kinetic** students who allow themselves the movement they need during study sessions report that during exams, they feel confident as they associate the material with the activity they used when they studied.

If you are **Oral/Aural,** add music to the work as well as to the background. Use a variety of tones and pitches as you recite the material. Singing otherwise boring lists of details will heighten your interest and facilitate your recollection of the items on the list. Think of childhood mnemonics for meaningless lists. Remember singing the ABC's or, your first brush with anatomy, "The head bone connected to the neck bone. . .?"

Round out your knowledge by adding the mental-function activities that are least natural for you. If you are a **Sensor**, create models and analogies. If you are an **Intuitive**, make lists and charts.

About Procrastination--The Emotional Warning Signals

Perceivers, fight your tendency to procrastinate. It's normal to avoid pain and to seek pleasure. When you feel insecure about material that makes you feel stupid, when you begin to have self-doubts, when you feel homesick or are physically ill, you may tend to put off studying.

Some students report that they procrastinate because they need to create a panic situation before they can get down to work. If this sounds like you, then ask yourself why this is so. Are you looking for external approval? Disapproval?

Sometimes negative feelings are so buried that you may not be aware that you *are* procrastinating. In these instances, catch yourself when you engage in such diversionary self-statements as: " I must clean my desk before I can sit down and study"; or "I'll get this phone call out of the way, then I'll be free to study uninterrupted"; or "I'll just cook some meals for the week, and I won't have to stop my studying to prepare dinner." There are untold ways in which you may be avoiding getting down to work. In the space below, write the delaying tactics that are *your* favorites.

When you find yourself engaged in time-wasting activities, STOP! *Schedule* a guilt-free session of no more than 20 minutes of delaying tactics, then spend 20 minutes with a comfortable subject that makes you feel secure. Once you're in the groove, you are ready to begin to tackle the more challenging material.

Notice the language of the above sentence. The word *challenging* replaces the negative word *difficult*. The use of positive self-talk will be discussed further in Chapter Six • Stress Management. Armed with insight and positive thoughts, you are now ready to enter the Optimal Memory Curve plan.

TIME ACCOUNTABILITY

Time Log and Time Pie

In order to create the best use of time--whether you are a **Sensing** or an **Intuitive** type--you will need to view time from two perspectives:

1. *Time Log,* using a **Sensing** linear representation
2. *Time Pie,* using an **Intuitive** model that shows patterns and proportions.

A Time Log reveals your time use in a segment-by-segment list fashion. This representation is preferred by **Sensing (S)** and **Judging (J)** types. Remember that **Sensing** types enjoy details and want data to appear sequentially. They prefer to orient themselves to the increments of time in the present. **Sensors** don't mind routine and schedules. **Judgers** depend on their need to plan, schedule, and come to closure.

A Time Pie shows a weekly pattern of time use. This spatial format allows **Intuitive (N)** types to represent time with their preference for patterns and analogies. The wedge-shaped visual pattern uses an analogy likening weekly time to a pie. N types tend to project themselves into the future. So that they can be fired by inspiration, **Intuitives** and **Perceivers** like to work with chunks of time rather than increments of time. N's and P's will tend to work around the clock when they are involved in an interesting subject or idea. They are inclined to lose sight of or to ignore schedules.

Remember to notice the time-gobblers that you try to overlook. Keep a written record of phone calls, mind wanderings, closet cleanings, trips to the refrigerator, and all the activities you engage in when you sabotage your efforts to study. Notice when you procrastinate, when you allow interruptions, and when you work at peak efficiency. Actually plan these activities into your guilt-free schedule. Whether you are a **Sensor** or an **Intuitive**, you will improve your time management if you use *both* the Time Log, incremental steps in the present, *and* the Time Pie, a more fluid projected time-use representation. By using both instruments, you will be able to accomplish manageable tasks each day and achieve your long-range goals.

Time Log Formulation

Keep a diary of your time use. Use a time chart or an appointment book to log each event. Apportion your time into 15-minute segments. Notice the time that you need to accomplish each task. Develop a conscious awareness of how long it takes you to bathe, prepare breakfast, make your bed (does anyone still do that?), exercise, walk to school. Construct optimal times based on your natural rhythms of energy peak and depletion. Reserve times of peak energy level for difficult tasks, and use your low energy level time for easy ones.

Adjust the example on the next page to begin with your wake-up time, and continue logging in hours until the time you retire.

TIME LOG

6.A.M._____	12:15_____
6:15_____	12:30_____
6:30_____	12:45_____
6:45_____	1:00_____
7:00_____	1:15_____
7:15_____	1:30_____
7:30_____	1:45_____
7:45_____	2:00_____
8:00_____	2:30_____
8:30_____	2:45_____
8:45_____	3:00_____
9:00_____	3:15_____
9:15_____	3:30_____
9:30_____	3:45_____
9:45_____	4:00_____
10:00_____	4:15_____
10:15_____	4:30_____
10:30_____	4:45_____
10:45_____	5:00_____
11:00_____	5:15_____
11:15_____	5:30_____
11:30_____	5:45_____
11:45_____	6:00_____
12:00_____	6:15_____

Use the space below to complete a 24-hour day.

_____
_____
_____
_____
_____
_____
_____
_____
_____
_____

   As you complete the time log, notice how much you are able to accomplish. Continue

this process throughout each 24-hour time segment for one week. Chart all of your waking

and sleeping hours.

Remember that a friendly attitude toward time use and momentary time lapses will help you to reach your goals. If you should awaken during the night and have difficulty getting back to sleep because you feel you must study, do what feels right to you. Rather than spend the time worrying, simply get up and study. You will catch up on sleep when you are less anxious. Chart the middle-of-night time as scheduled study time, accepting it as productive antianxiety action time rather than disturbed sleep time.

Don't punish yourself if you daydream. Daydreaming and "goofing off," if kept under control, can be viewed as refreshing interludes. Remember that the creative, time-efficient composer Beethoven said, "Rests are also music."

Time Pie

Once you have accounted for your time in your Time Log, you are ready to represent your time in chunks. Slice the time pie in sections corresponding to the time you think you need for each of the items below:

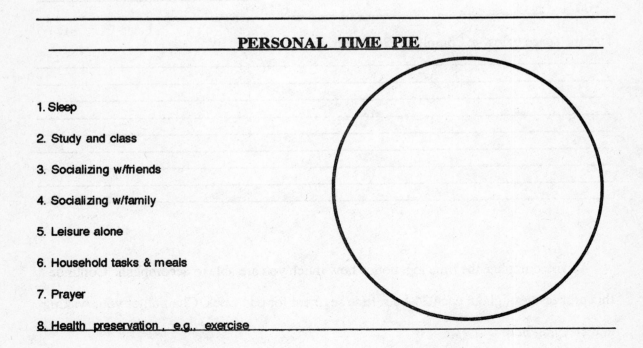

PERSONAL TIME PIE

1. Sleep

2. Study and class

3. Socializing w/friends

4. Socializing w/family

5. Leisure alone

6. Household tasks & meals

7. Prayer

8. Health preservation , e.g., exercise

Tabulate your time based on a seven-day week. Think about how you use segments of time. Do you need eight hours' sleep daily? If so, use one third of the pie for sleep, item #1.

<u>To succeed in exams, you must devote at least two hours of independent study for each hour of class time.</u> So if you spend four hours in class, you will need eight hours of independent study, for a total of 12 hours, or one half of the time pie for item #2.

Now divide the remainder of the time into wedges that correspond to the other areas of your life that need attention. Notice that not much time is left for anything other than the bare essentials.

The trick to efficient time use is to combine tasks. For example, household tasks (#6) can be accomplished while you socialize with friends or family (#3 and #4).

Physical exercise can be combined with rote memorization. Some students find that listening to a taped lecture while bike riding releases tension and reinforces memory.

Use the space below to write the tasks that you might combine to save time.

Below is the time pie of a successful second-year medical student, Student ß. This represents her time expenditure in the two weeks before National Boards.

PERSONAL TIME PIE: Student ß

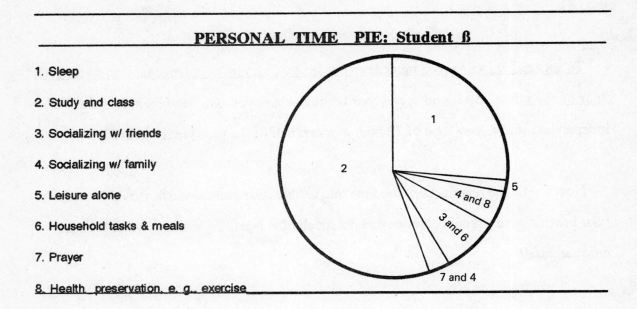

1. Sleep

2. Study and class

3. Socializing w/ friends

4. Socializing w/ family

5. Leisure alone

6. Household tasks & meals

7. Prayer

8. Health preservation, e. g., exercise

It's important that you make your time do double duty so that you have enough time to complete your goals. Notice the combining of #3 and #6; #4 and #8; #7 and #4 . Study can be more fun in the company of friends (combining #2 and #3.)

You need the support of your loved ones. You will get that support if people you care about understand what you are doing. If they feel excluded, folks you would want to count on can unconsciously sabotage you in your time-management efforts. For this reason, give close buddies a copy of your Time Log and Time Pie. Ask them to help you manage your time.

Once family, friends, and lovers see your schedule, they will understand why you are not as available to them as they would like. This will give them the opportunity to help you even if they don't enjoy being deprived of time with you. You don't need a fight or a guilt-producing episode just before an exam, so plan ahead to balance your school goals with your personal needs.

STUDY TRICKS AND TREATS
Methods for Time Efficiency

Sandwich subjects you dislike between two slices of those that you enjoy. Tackle difficult areas when you are refreshed. Treat yourself to your favorite subjects only when you have finished a section of the nasties.

Give yourself small rewards as you complete a challenging task. If your reward is to talk on the telephone, keep the call pleasant and monitor its length.

If you need an hour break to enjoy a special TV program, take it. When the program ends, turn off the TV. Those who have a hard time leaving the television set can get some help from the hardware store. Plug your TV into an electrical outlet timer so that it disconnects immediately after your program. That will do the dirty work for you

In the space below, write your favorite ways of taking mini-breaks from your studies.

We all have reasons for missing work. In the space below, list situations that cause you to fall behind in your work. What can you do to correct the time-eaters?

Catching Up with Missed Work

If you fall behind in your studies (and you will), keep the memory curve high by working on the *most current* material *before* attempting to make up lost work. If you didn't have time to study on Monday and Tuesday, and here it is Wednesday, read, label, chart, and reinforce Wednesday's work. Do Thursday's work on Thursday, Friday's work on Friday. When the weekend comes, make up the missed work of Monday and Tuesday. If you continually try to play catch-up, you will always feel guilty, inadequate, or flustered as if entering the middle of a movie.

SUMMARY

Save time and create an active system for reinforcing your memory. The time-efficient study methods that work include the following steps.

1. Look! Before attending class, skim read your textbook, scanning the text for bold-face, italics, and special print, charts, pictures, and diagrams. Attend to tables of contents and to summary statements in order to develop a glossary of unfamiliar terms. After class, use a variety of writing styles and colors to label and organize your notes.

2. Listen! Attend class and listen for the pitches and tones used by the lecturer as she presents the material. The emphasis expressed in the music of her voice will help you to identify the important points for further study. Repeat the material aloud as soon as you can speak after class. Hear yourself sounding confident.

3. Move! Get physically involved. Write the material as you hear it in the lecture. Use an in-the-ear, out-the hand method of note taking, attempting to capture all data. If you can't write fast enough, skip a space and move on. Fill in the blanks when you review data

at home. At home, rewrite the material on a chalkboard or on large paper tacked to your wall. In this way, you will use large muscles as you reinforce your learning through movement.

4. Analyze! Label your notes. What are the Requirements for a process to proceed? What are the Steps of the process? Where is the bifurcation? The merging? Why? What are the Results in terms of Cause and Effect? Ask "What would happen if . . .?" questions. Suppose some required step in the process were missing? What then might the results be? How do Structure, Function, and Mechanism of Action interrelate?

5. Synthesize! How does this information fit with what you already know? What are the possible clinical implications?

6. Integrate! Go over the information as you walk, jog, or dance through your daily chores. Use your body to make the material live in your bones.

7. Say! Talk about the material with your colleagues. Teach the material to others. The best way to learn is to teach. If you have no other person to teach, teach the material to your coffee cup.

8. Organize! Set short-range and long-range goals. Time is the precious stuff that life is made of. Use time wisely. To kill time is to murder your opportunity for success.

References

Adler, T.(1991) Cumulative learning aids memory. *The APA Monitor* 22 (2), pp 10-11

Alpert, R. and Haber, R. N. (1960) Anxiety in academic achievement situations. *Journal of Abnormal Social Psychology,* 61 pp 207-215

Bellezza, F.S. (1981) Mnemonic devices, classification, characteristics, and criteria. *Review of Educational Research,* 51, pp 247-275

Bower, G.H. and Bolton, L.S. (1969) Why are rhymes easy to learn? *Journal of Experimental Psychology,* 82, pp 453-461

Canaday, S.D. and Lancaster, C.J. (1985) Impact of undergraduate courses on medical students' performance in basic sciences. *Journal of Medical Education,* 60 pp 757-763

Houle, C. (1984) *Patterns of Learning.* San Francisco: Jossey-Bass Pub

Montecinos, C. and Jackson, E.W. (1987) Metacognitive factors affecting performance on MCAT skills analysis: Reading practice passages. *Proceedings of the Twenty-Sixth Annual Conference Research in Medical Education* Wash., D.C., Association of American Medical Colleges pp 63-68

Shain, D.D. and Kelliher, G. J. (1988) A study skills workshop as an integral part of orientation to medical school: The establishment of self-directed learning *Proceedings of the Twenty-Seventh Annual Conference Research in Medical Education* Chicago, Il, Association of American Medical Colleges pp 91-96

Sims, W.L. (1980) *The effect of pitch and rhythm on the short-term memorization of nonsense syllable sequences by college students.* Unpublished master's thesis, Kent State University.

Weinert, F. E. and Perlmutter, M., Editors (1988) *Memory Development: Universal Changes and Individual Differences.* Hillside, NJ: Erlbaum Assoc

Wolf, F.M., Ulman, J.G., Slatman, G.A., and Savickas, M.L. (1980) Allocation of time
and perceived coping behavior of first-year medical students. *Journal of Medical
Education,* 56 pp 956-958

Suggested Readings

Cermak, L. S. and Craik, F. I. M., Editors (1979) *Levels of Processing in Human
Memory.* Hillside, NJ: Erlbaum Associates

Macan, T. H. , Shahani, C., Dipboye, R. L., and Phillips, A. P. (1990) College students'
time management: Correlations with academic performance and stress. *Journal of
Educational Psychology,* 82 (4) pp760-768

Neisser, U. and Winograd, E., Editors (1988) *Remembering Reconsidered.*
N.Y: Cambridge University Press

Shain, D. D. (1989) Self-directed learning and collegial interaction through the
use of the Myers-Briggs Type Indicator in medical education. In *Proceedings APT
VIII Biennial International Conference, Boulder CO Frontiers of Psychological
Type* Gainsville, FL Association for Psychological Type pp 101-104

CHAPTER THREE • TAKING NOTES

There are two good reasons for taking notes. One is to create your own text, and the other is to help you to stay active and awake in class. Education research indicates that students who take notes "tend to emphasize and remember important information and discard the less important information" (Kiewra et al., 1991) and that "learning depends upon the capacity for attention, as well as the related function of concentration" (Cohler, 1989). Your notes will become your primary study textbook. Once you have organized the notes, you will use them to determine what's important and what is not.

Purpose

This chapter will provide you with techniques designed to produce an organized and efficient system of note-taking. By the end of this chapter, you will be able to use your notes to test your breadth and depth of understanding, and you will be able to improve your note-taking skills in the following situations:

1. taking classroom notes--an auditory to visual process
2. labeling notes--an analytic/organizational, decision-making process
3. taking textbook notes--a visual to analytic and memorization process
4. organizational components--an integrating process.

TAKING CLASSROOM NOTES

Unless the professor uses a Socratic questioning method to actively involve students, most medical school lectures consist of a deluge of details presented rapidly, with little time for you to analyze the data. You spend most of your time as a passive recipient of an instructor's idea of what is relevant. Active learners who use all their senses learn more than passive spectators. We know that "knowledge is not something that can be obtained passively from the outside world but has to be *actively constructed*. . . in accordance with the searchlight theory of the mind" (Anthony, 1989).

Note-taking helps you to become an active analyst. Some students prefer just to sit and listen to a lecture. They say they have trouble understanding the lecture if they try to write what is being said. Because the spoken word is elusive, simply listening will not give you a permanent record of the important details of the lecture. Although it may be true that while you are taking notes you cannot analyze what is being said, full understanding will take place after class as you organize your notes. Remember that one of the goals of note-taking is to gather information for later organization, and you will overcome problems with in-class concentration.

Classroom Note-Taking Necessities

To put together comprehensive notes, space and speed are essential. Leave a two-inch margin, and use only one side of the page. Arm yourself with lots of three-ring loose-leaf paper, some comfortable-to-hold pens, and a clipboard, and secure whatever seating arrangement will enhance rapid writing. Nylon-tipped pens are best for taking your class notes because they glide without much friction resistance.

Write as much as you possibly can. Adopt an in-the-ear, out-the-hand attitude. Do not stop to ponder the material while you write. Abbreviate, leave out vowels, invent symbols to take the place of words. I have included a list of some suggested symbols at the end of this chapter.

While whizzing through your writing , if you get lost (and you will), skip a space and move on. Pick up your writing when you catch on. Don't worry about getting behind in your note-taking. Getting lost is valuable information about what you know and what you don't. Empty spaces will usually occur immediately after a word or concept that you didn't understand. You will fill in the gaps later.

Some students become embarrassed if they don't understand something that they think they should know, so they leave holes in their notes. These folks tend to be independent types who prefer to ferret out information on their own, but despite their good intentions, the pressure of time causes them to leave questions in the notes unanswered. Don't allow yourself to tolerate blank spaces. You may intend to get back to them, but because of time constraints, you probably won't. *Unanswered questions create insecurity and cause t ime-consuming gaps in your understanding.*

To avoid gaps in gathering information, select a reliable note-taking partner. The best note-taking partner is someone of a complementary and opposite learning-style type. If you have identified yourself as **Intuitive**, select a **Sensor**. If you are a **Sensor**, find an **Intuitive** as your buddy.

At the end of the lecture, *before you gather your books and leave the room*, fill in blank spaces. Ask your note-taking partner for any information you might have missed. If you are both baffled, ask the professor to clarify your uncertainties. If the professor is unavailable, or if you came to class unprepared and feel unable to ask an intelligent question, ferret out the information from graduate students in the department, from textbooks, from slides kept on file in the library, from a tutor, or through any other creative method you can devise.

LABELING NOTES

All exam questions are based on *labels*. Labels are subheadings, or identifying words that organize clusters of details that affect or relate to one another. Labels help you to make associations and solve problems. The labels you select will aid you in recall of the details and the concepts you need to analyze data.

To take advantage of the optimal memory curve, write your labels in the margins of your classroom notes within the first 24 hours after class. Use a different writing style or another color to make the labels stand out.

If you use pencil for your initial labeling, you will be able to change the labels when you think of better ones. The analytic process of deciding which label to use helps you to manage, categorize, and remember large amounts of random details. Once you have decided on the best labels, you can use them to construct flash cards and charts.

Labels become the titles at the top of each column of your chart. The example that follows will demonstrate the use of labels in an anatomy chart. If you want exercise in using the chart, fill in the details that fit under each label.

GROSS ANATOMY: BONES

Bone Types	Characteristics						
	Class	Development	Location	Visual Identifiers			
				Skeleton /	Picture /	Lab /	X-ray

Now create a similar chart showing *characteristics* of the Joints, indicating *Types of Joints, Class of Joints*--synarthrosis, amphiarthrosis, and diarthrosis--*Location, Movements, Blood Supply,* and *Nerve Supply.*

Construct a chart for muscles, showing *Types of muscles, Location, Attachments, Origin, Insertion, Function, Action, Blood Supply,* and *Nerve Supply.*

Notice that because use of the word *characteristic* is too broad, we have used more specific sublabels below that word on the chart. For labels to be valuable as memory pegs for exams, you will want to create labels that are as specific and narrowly defined as possible. For clarity, the label characteristics is refined to include a series of specific labels related to *limited characteristics*, such as: *location, size, shape, color, texture, smell, type, blood supply, nerve supply, chemical properties, physical properties, normal values, anomalies.*

Labels or subheadings related to mechanisms and process courses such as physiology, biochemistry, pathology, and pharmacology would include specific identifying words.

A list of these words follows.

Mechanical and Chemical Processes	*Primary/Secondary*
Method and Mechanism of Action	*Acute/Chronic*
Requirements	*Significance*
Results in terms of Cause and Effect	*Rules and Principles*
Specific Steps and Number of Steps	*Types*
Direction of the Process	*Analogies*
Chemical and/or Physical Components	*Examples*
Action/Reaction	*Clinical implications*
Course of Action/Reaction	*Symptoms*
Circumstances of Action/Reaction	*Diagnosis*
Duration of Action/Reaction	*Treatment*

You can add to your vocabulary of labels as you begin to sort out your notes.

In physical objects courses, the labels or subheadings related to the concrete aspects of the anatomy of an organ would include such buzzwords, or labels, as: *Structure, Function, Mechanism of Action, Location, Origin, Development, Morphology, Definition, Composition, Clinical Implications, Components, Types.* Specific *characteristics* include: *appearance, size, shape, color, smell, texture.* Always add labels that specify distinguishing details: *Compare/Contrast; Similarities/Differences ...*

By organizing an otherwise disorganized batch of details under their label subheadings, you develop your ability to analyze the data. Once the data are analyzed, you can make decisions about them and begin to organize a large amount of material into smaller, manageable packages of information to be memorized (Willey and Jarecky, 1976).

In addition to multiple-choice examinations, some courses use essay writing as a means of evaluating your depth of understanding. Labels are the organizing landmarks in good essays. When you are asked to define or describe, you will include the labels related to *category, origin, function, location*. List specific characteristics such as *appearance, size, shape, color, texture*.

In physical objects courses, include *composition, structure*, and the *physical* and *chemical components*. In process courses, state the *origin, method/mechanism, location, steps, roles requirements, results* in terms of *cause and effect*.

When you are asked to *discuss* a topic, start your essay with the labels you used to define and describe. Expand the essay by adding information corresponding to your *compare/contrast* labels. List examples, giving the specific characteristics inherent in each example.

Using Labels to Construct Exam Questions

To integrate your study efforts, be sure to add possible examination questions to the end of each section of your notes. Use labels to create the stem of the question. The following example is a clinical case study question:

A 20 old woman presents with cardiac concerns. On examination you discover a midsystolic click. What possible diagnosis will you consider. Why? What other findings will you look for to corroborate your diagnosis?

In the space below, construct your own question related to the cardiac system.

Expanding Class Notes

Use the blank page facing your notes to fill in information from your textbook, from handouts, and from discussions with colleagues. Your notes represent your understanding of what is important about the lecture. Additional information can be enhancing or clarifying. To distinguish the notes you took in class from information you got from another source, use a different colored ink. This is especially important if you are a visual learner.

When you are pressed to recall information during exams, you will be able to close your eyes and *see* the labels you wrote in different colors. You will be able mentally to place those items that stand out on the left or right page as you remember your labels and their corresponding details.

Leaving Space

Leave ample room for development of your notes. The cheapest thing in medical school is paper. Don't be afraid to write large and give yourself plenty of room for expansion. Don't try to cram additions into small spaces above or below your class notes. On the blank facing page, add possible exam questions, diagrams, charts, and clinical correlations to the basic information.

When your notes are thorough and complete, you can work with them as your primary examination review book throughout your tenure as a medical student and refer to them when you are an intern and a resident.

TAKING TEXTBOOK NOTES

In preparation for examinations, you will, in addition to your classroom notes, read, analyze, and review textbooks. These books will give you the supplemental material you need to enrich your personal text of lecture and lab notes. Be sure to read tables of contents, introductory paragraphs, and summary statements at the end of each chapter.

The value of the notes you make from your reading will depend on your skill at determining which things to copy from textbooks, which information to skim, how fast you can write, and when and how to time your note-taking. To develop your critical- thinking capacity, be organized in your reading and note-taking.

ORGANIZATIONAL COMPONENTS
Headings

Headings appear at the top of the body of information. They help you to keep organized by telling you what you will be reading about. They tend to be the broad titles. For example, a typical heading might be *Cardiac System*. Because headings are so obvious, **Intuitive** students often tend to make the mistake of overlooking them.

Details and Items

The details and items are the running narratives, the collections of facts. Details give the material depth and significance. Some details may be extraneous, nonessential information. If the details are related to structure, function, and mechanism of action, or if you can add a label to the details, they are probably important. **Sensing** types usually enjoy details; **Intuitive** types tend not to pay enough attention to them.

The details and items included under the heading *Cardiac System* would encompass all the information related to the developmental, cellular, anatomic, physiologic, biochemical, electrical, pathological, pharmacological, historical, and clinical aspects of the cardiac system.

Labels

Labels, as we discussed before, are the concepts, subheadings, or identifying words that organize clusters of details that affect or relate to one another. They tell you why and in what way the details are important. In the cardiac system, the labels would relate to the *structure* of the heart, its *function,* its *mechanism of action,* the *results* in terms of *cause and effect* of other organ systems that affect the heart . . . and all characteristics we have already listed in the section about labeling notes.

Labeling Textbooks

As you read professionally written textbooks, if you are like most medical students you undoubtedly use bright-colored markers to accent significant information. Why do you create these visual highlights? Is it because you feel that the information is important? Do you highlight areas that are unclear? Do you plan to return to the material for further clarification and review? All of these reasons are fine! But be realistic: you probably won't have time to get back to this material.

If you want to remember the highlighted stuff, you need to do some active analysis. Give the highlighting significance by adding a *label* to the margin of your highlighted material. Let's work together to demonstrate adding labels to a passage in a text.

In the example on the following page, taken from page 72 of the Oklahoma Notes, *Pathology,* we have an information sample, Mitral Valve Prolapse. Notice the labels I have added to the margin. Having taken the time to add labels to your text, you can discover what you remember by covering the information sample on the right and answering questions that the labels suggest.

III Mitral Valve Prolapse - Common condition (5-7% of

Incidence   general   population, most frequently young women) which may in

Origin   some cases be congenital in origin.

Symptoms   Characterized by enlarged mitral leaflets, elongated chordae, or

Results   both. This allows for ballooning of leaflet during systole and may

Effect   produce a midsystolic click corresponding to the snapping of an

Sound   everted leaflet. . . ."

In your notebook, you can add some sample examination questions, like those that follow.

What is the incidence of mitral valve prolapse?

What is the origin of the disorder?

How does mitral valve prolapse present clinically?

What symptoms might you expect to find?

What sounds result from a prolapsed mitral valve?

Examinations may use a vocabulary different from yours, so to anticipate every possible exam question, think of synonyms for any labels you find within the body of the text. The concept of the label, incidence, could also be implied with words like *occurrence, population, epidemiology, etiology. Origin* might be labeled *cause. Symptoms* might also be called *clinical findings.* It is not important which label you choose. What is important is that you have thought about the material and used an identifying word as a memory peg. This memory peg will become your access word for recall of the data.

When you are organizing your notes at home, use colored pens to coordinate the labels. Mark them with consistent abbreviations. For example, for *Structure*, you might write *St* in green: for *Function* write *Fxn* in red: for *Mechanism of Action*, *MA* in brown.

Once you develop a color-coded system and a vocabulary of labels, when confronted with the label in an exam question you will be able to picture it and remember the details related to it in your textbook and in your notes. You will gain confidence as you meet the identifying labeling words. Remember that in all exam questions, the labels are the pivotal words.

Indented Format

When you take notes from textbooks, use an indented format on the page facing your handwritten classroom notes. This configuration will help you to specify headings, labels, and details from which to study and to formulate examination questions.

When you use a methodical system of gathering information from a textbook into a concise, indented format, you will not need to gather an entire library on your desk for further review or reference. When preparing for exams, instead of juggling an unmanageable pile of textbooks, you will find that having all your study materials in one comprehensive self-written volume will save you time and will give you the security that comes from being organized.

There are four steps to follow to achieve an indented format organization. They are:

1. Determine the topic.

2. Write the topic at the top of the page.

3. Use labels as subheadings, selecting the specific label from those you have

   placed in the margins of your textbook.

4. Add only relevant and necessary details under the label subheadings.

In the space below, construct indented format notes from the following information sample.

	III Mitral Valve Prolapse - Common condition (5-7% of general
Incidence	population, most frequently young women) which may in some
Origin	cases be congenital in origin.
Symptoms	Characterized by enlarged mitral leaflets, elongated chordae, or
Results	both. This allows for ballooning of leaflet during systole and may
Effect	produce a midsystolic click corresponding to the snapping of an
Sound	everted leaflet. . . ."

Does yours look something like the following example?

Cardiac System

PATHOLOGY

Valvular Diseases

Mitral Valve Prolapse

Incidence

Common 5-7% pop.

young women

Origin

congenital

Symptom Characterization

enlarged mitral leaflets (either or both)

elongated chordae

Results

ballooning of leaflet--during systole

Clinical Findings

Sound

midsystolic click--snapping of everted leaflet

Chart Construction and Use

Remember that we used labels to organize the charts into headings and subheadings. Now let's pay attention to concise formatting. When organizing your notes, condense the material into convenient-to-carry cell charts or flow charts. If you carry your charts with you, you can use them when you might otherwise waste time: when you are stuck in traffic or in line at the bank. Daily chart use helps you to attain long-term memory of details. With charts, the challenge of studying for National Boards becomes a routine exercise in review rather than a panic-driven agony.

Cell Chart

The example that follows was derived from the Oklahoma Notes, *Gross Anatomy*, page 42. The material was presented in indented format. Let's create a cell chart.

THE LEG: LATERAL COMPARTMENT

COMPONENTS

	Muscles	Bones	Tendons	Joints
Location				
Origin				
Insertion				
Function				
Action				
Nerve Supply				
Blood Supply				

Fill in the chart above and add to it any other data that you feel are missing.

Refer to the chart and draw the lateral compartment of the leg.

Were you able to visualize all the components? Can you name the parts from memory?

<u>Flow Chart</u>

The following simple flow chart is found on page 84, Fig. 3-4, of the Oklahoma Notes, *Physiology.* When you use a flow chart, add as you proceed, the labels: requirements, steps, number of steps, direction of steps, action/reaction, results/cause/effect.

Cardiac Output

<u>The multiple factors that determine cardiac output</u>

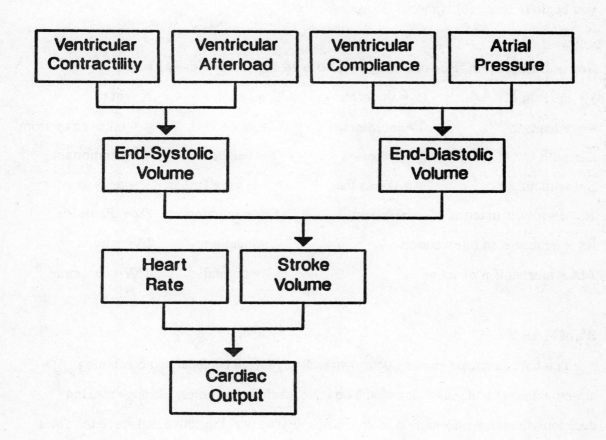

Can you see that using this handy way of visualizing large amounts of information gives you a concise reference for thorough review?

Similarities and differences are favorite components in examination questions. So when you create charts, pay particular attention to similarities and differences. Place compare/contrast data next to each. Notice the aspects of sizes, shapes, functions, and mechanisms of action in data that have many variables in common but some differentiating features. The ability to discriminate between minor differences challenges your ability to be a skillful detective, a necessary talent for the discerning clinician.

After each course examination, add to your notes a section that includes all the concepts and facts you missed on the exam. This compilation of weak areas will be invaluable when you begin to study for National Boards.

Some Suggested "Shorthand" Symbols to Speed Note-Taking

Σ = the sum of	$\therefore$ = therefore	$U/$ = usually	N = not
$\rightarrow$ = leads to	$\uparrow$ = increases	$\male$ = male	$\Leftarrow$ = takes away from
$\bar{C}$ = with	$\downarrow$ = decreases	$\female$ = female	! * = important
$\bar{S}$ = without	< = is less than	> = is greater than	+ = adds to
$R/c\text{-}e$ = results in terms of cause/effect		Fxn = function	Dx = diagnosis
Rx = treatment or intervention		L = location	$?\text{?}$ = why
MA = mechanism of action		$N/$ = normal	AbN = abnormal

SUMMARY

You have practiced creating your own well-organized personal text combining classroom notes and textbook notes. You have labeled your notes. Through making decisions about the information in your notes, you've become active and made the notes meaningful and memorable. You have created charts of the important data and have combined your auditory, visual, and intellectual capacities. You are ready to move on to apply your learning to the problem-solving exercises in the next chapter.

References

Anthony, E. J. (1989) The psychoanalytic approach to learning theory (with more than a passing reference to Piaget). In *Learning and Education: Psychoanalytic Perspectives* Eds. Field, K., Cohler, B., and Wool, G. Madison, CT: International Universities Press Inc pp 99-125

Cohler, B. (1989) Psychoanalysis and education: Motive, meaning, and self. In *Learning and Education: Psychoanalytic Perspectives*. Eds. Field, K., Cohler, B. and Wool, G. Madison, CT: International Universities Press Inc pp 11-68.

Kiewra, K. A., Mayer, R. E., Christensen, M., Kim, S., and Risch, N. (1991) Effects of repetition on recall and notetaking; Strategies for learning from lectures *Journal of Educational Psychology* 83 (1) pp120-123

Willey, M. and Jarecky, B. (1976) *Analysis and Application of Information.* Developed at Howard University College of Medicine and University of Kentucky College of Dentistry

CHAPTER FOUR   •   PROBLEM-SOLVING

We solve problems every day. The problems can range from the simple act of changing a light bulb to the more challenging dilemmas of foreign affairs and biomedical science. Every time you meet a patient, you will become a professional problem-solver. But,before you can begin to take care of a patient's illness, you must know what the problem is.

This involves using a multistep problem-solving process that combines *what is* and *what might be*. Thus, theory combines with practice as you see the patient through educated eyes. Once the patient and his symptoms have been carefully observed, you can proceed to deduce the probable causes of the illness. Your study and test-taking regimen as a medical student will help you to get ready for the problem-solving skills you will need as a physician.

Purpose

The purpose of this chapter is to identify and apply the five basic steps you need to solve problems individually and in groups.

These steps will ask you to:

• know yourself and expand your learning-style techniques

• define the problem

• devise a strategy or plan of attack by establishing subgoals

• execute the strategy

• evaluate your progress toward the goal

KNOW YOURSELF

How do you solve problems? Consider the steps you take. Learning theorists tell us that problem-solving is a learned skill. They have found that the problem-solving prerequisites--memory, time, processing capacity, motivation, flexibility, control of goal direction, simple discrimination learning, and recognition of complexities--are essential in the learner if problem-solving is to occur. Confronted with a problem, the learner must apply rules for problem-solving (Wilhite, 1990).

Individual Differences in Problem-Solving Skills

Have you ever wondered why some people can solve problems easily and others cannot? The question has long interested psychologists and educators. "Any complete answer to this question, as a minimum, will necessarily involve specification of specific problem solving competencies *(content)*, an understanding of underlying psychological mechanisms *(cognition)*, and some way to deal with *individual differences*" (Scandura, 1977).

Content—A body of knowledge must be available. This knowledge must be readily available or retrievable from memory. Memorized material is retrievable when knowledge has been reinforced immediately after new material is learned and at intermittent intervals over time.

Cognition--As a successful problem-solver, you will need to understand the meaning of the problem statement. What is actually being asked? In the case of a simple problem, like deciding to change a light bulb when a lamp goes dark, you will usually rule out possible causes of the problem before you take action.

Although problem-solving skills can be taught and learned, the problem-solver must be intellectually and emotionally equipped to think clearly. *Individual differences in physiological capacities and generalized physical and intellectual maturation and endowment will determine whether or not a person can solve problems logically.*

As a medical student under pressure, you have by now discovered that your problem- solving skills can vary with course content and with how you happen to be feeling. The presence or absence of unresolved emotional conflicts can have a profound effect on your problem-solving capacities. Previous educational exposure to experiences that afford practice with problem-solving techniques can stack the deck for or against you.

Negative internal or external influences aside, you can train yourself to define and solve problems by taking steps that break down the problem into its logical components. First you will need to observe what is; then you will devise a hypothesis.

In the example of the possibly dead bulb, your reasoning goes something like this: The light doesn't work. Why? Is the lamp plugged into a live socket? Is the switch turned on? If the answer to both these questions is yes, then you work on the *assumption* that the bulb is burned out. You unscrew the bulb, look for damage, shake it and listen for a broken filament. The bulb makes a rattling sound, so you replace it with a new one. Voilà! If your premise about the cause of the darkness was correct, light appears.

Expand Learning-Style Techniques

Your learning-style strengths and limitations can help or hinder your ability to solve problems. Your natural problem-solving steps are determined by your individual learning style and by your previous experiences with solving problems. As you remember from Chapter One • Learning Styles, the methods you use to take in information and make decisions about information are based on your preference for **Sensing** or **Intuition**, **Thinking** or **Feeling**.

By way of a quick review, the mental functions can be characterized as follows:

Sensing--knowing what is

Thinking--understanding meanings

Intuition--envisioning what might be

Feeling--knowing the value of things

Regardless of your inborn learning-style preference, you will need to develop and use all four mental functions: **Sensing**, **Intuition**, **Thinking**, and **Feeling**. Problem solutions can be complete only when the steps encompass *details* **(S)** and *concepts* **(N)**, *objectivity* **(T)** and *subjectivity* **(F)**.

"In order to avoid confusion while solving problems, the problem-solver will need to follow a systematic process which uses only one mental process at a time. The four mental functions *Sensing, Intuition, Thinking,* and *Feeling* will be used sequentially, consciously, and with purpose" (McCaulley 1987). After you have worked on the problem by using the four mental functions sequentially, you will complete your work through the use of *Extraversion, Introversion, Judging,* and *Perceiving.* Let's go through the steps together, and then we'll apply them to your methods of studying and test-taking.

Using Sensing, Intuition, Thinking, and Feeling

1. Use **Sensing** to observe the details inherent in the problem: What is here for you to observe now? Because **Sensing** establishes what exists in the present, the **Sensing** perception focuses on using all your senses to discern immediate experiences, acute powers of observation, memory for details, and practicality.

In the case of the problem with the light bulb, you don't need to be a genius to notice that you are sitting in the dark. You try to solve the problem by switching on the light. The switch clicks, but the lamp does not produce light. From these *observable facts*, you know that there is a problem. Your observations lead you to the next step: "Why?"

In the case of studying about a biomedical problem, let's say a malfunction of an anatomic structure, you follow the same procedure, but your observations are more encompassing. You observe a *normal* structure and its components as they exist in the present. What do you see, feel, smell, and hear? Notice the size, shape, color, appearance, composition, viscosity, density, cell types, physical properties, chemical properties, scope, and limits of this structure. What is the relationship of this structure and its parts with other contiguous structures?

You pay attention to similarities and dissimilarities of this structure to other structures. In your observations, you compare and contrast, form an internal visual representation, and follow an orderly progression of steps while viewing the structure. You look from outer to inner surfaces, from left to right, from top to bottom. You notice all the facts of what *is*, not what might be, in this initial step. Once you have understood *normal* values, now you are ready to ask about the causes of the malfunction of this structure.

2. Use **Intuition** to seek patterns, develop new possibilities, and formulate a hypothesis. Remember that the **Intuitive** process of perceiving refers to perceptions of possibilities, meanings, and relationships.

Again, back to the light bulb: Why didn't the light work? You ran through your observations--it's dark. Then you began to ask why. Even in the initial observation stage, you looked for cause-effect relationships. "Is the lamp plugged in? Is the switch in the 'on' position? Once you checked these out and found nothing else wrong, you began to define the problem by *assuming* that it was with the bulb.

In anticipating a solution to any problem, you will ask, "What would happen if . . .?" In the light bulb case, in order to determine that the problem is the bulb and not the electrical outlet, you might ask, "What would happen if I plugged another lamp into this outlet? Would it work?"

In biomedical problem situations, you must always go beyond *what is* to include *what might be*. **Intuitive** perceptions may come to the surface as a sudden recognition of a pattern or relationship in seemingly unrelated events. An **Intuitive** perceiver looks for patterns and projects perceptions into the future. As a competent problem-solver, you must include the **Intuitive** function and ask yourself more complex questions related to cause and effect.

When you study normal values, you must amplify your knowledge by anticipating problem situations. For example, in studying the information about an anatomical structure, in addition to using your **Sensing** powers of observation, you must engage your **Intuitive** self by asking: "What would happen if the structure changes? How might that affect the function? What changes might occur in the mechanism of action?" In problem solving related to a biochemical process, you might ask: "If X is the normal value, what would happen if X changes?" You hypothesize about relationships: "If the *cause* changes, how will the *results* change? If these are the requirements for a process to proceed, what would happen if the requirements were increased, were decreased, or were not present?"

To apply any basic science subject to medicine, go beyond a mere acceptance of what is. Develop a problem-solving study format by asking "What would happen if . . .?" questions, look for patterns and interrelationships. What might you expect? Develop a hypothesis (Wessells, 1982).

Use the following questions as guides in your hypothesis formulation:

• After you observe *what is*, ask yourself, *what might be?*

• What functions do the shapes imply?

• What are the shapes analogous to?

• Based on its flexibility and texture, how durable is the structure?

• Based on the viscosity of the fluid, the bends in the path of flow, and the size of the openings, how might the velocity of flow be affected?

• How do pressure and speed interrelate?

3. Use **Thinking** to make an objective analysis of the situation. What are the *guiding principles*? Have you considered all options? Step back from the question and your answer to take an objective look. How might you view the situation differently? Look at cause and effect, consequences, alternatives.

In the case of the light bulb, you do not curse the dark or complain about the person who let the light burn all night. You remain *objective* and evaluate what needs to be done. Can you buy another bulb? If not, can you snitch one from another lamp, which you are not using? Your **Thinking** function tells you: don't fret about it; find a solution.

During the problem-solving process in an exam, you should not curse the examiner, nor is it helpful to complain that the problem is unfair. Step back. Look for guiding principles. Notice the internal logic of the exam questions. **Thinking** relies on *objective* principles of cause-effect, and links ideas together by making logical connections.

4. After you have completed the first three steps, **Sensing**, **Intuition**, and **Thinking**, you are ready to take the fourth step and ask yourself if your subjective view of the problem *feels* right to you. Use your natural gift of **Feeling** to determine how deeply you care about your choice. In making your *subjective* evaluation, put more weight on usual rather than unusual occurrences, on permanent rather than temporary effects. In the final analysis, as a physician, only you can be accountable for your decisions, so trust your well-informed opinion.

Using Extraversion and Introversion, Judging and Perceiving

You have worked alone using all four mental function steps, and now you are ready to amplify your understanding. The steps you take will expand your preferred energy source--**Extraversion** or **Introversion**--and your decision-making capacity-- **Judging** or **Perceiving**.

1. Use **Extraversion** to clarify your ideas with others. Find people who have more information than you do. These may be people you know--a teacher, a fellow student, a personal acquaintance--or may exist only in written texts.

When you talk with others about the problem, use the mental-function steps in order: **Sensing, Intuition, Thinking,** and **Feeling.** You might say something to the effect: "I observe . . ., therefore I suppose that . . . I think . . .," and finally, "I feel . . ." When baffled by a problem, students often make the mistake of starting with "I feel . . ." and get bogged down by self-defeating subjectivity.

2. Use **Introversion** and go off by yourself to think deeply about the problem. Follow the steps **Sensing**, **Intuitive**, **Thinking**, and **Feeling** in order.

3. Use **Perceiving** to be sure you have considered all reasonable and available data and possibilities related to the problem. Remember to attend to details as they exist in the present, but do not stay locked in the present. Look over your shoulder and expand your view as you consider what-would-happen-if . . .? possibilities.

4. Use **Judgment** to stay on track. Try not to be diverted to side issues. Adhere to a realistic time schedule. Once you have as much information as you need, come to closure and move on.

Now that you have practiced expanding your learning style, you are ready to tackle the problem. The following problem-solving steps will keep you organized and on track.

DEFINE THE PROBLEM

You cannot solve a problem until you know what the problem is. To define the problem accurately, you must understand the language of the problem statement. In problem-solving examination questions, ask yourself: What words are used? What does each word mean?

To be sure that you are clear about what is being asked, look carefully at the verbs and at the qualifying words that narrow the focus of the problem--age, sex, location, origin.

If the question is long and complicated, break it into phrases and determine what each phrase means. If the problem is related to a structure or a biochemical process, observe what is there for you to see. From what you can observe and from what you know about normal values of that structure or process, what aspect of the structure or process is the problem related to?

Some problem statements are clearer than others. An easy-to-define problem has a starting point and an achievable goal. Problems that are difficult to define often lack discernible starting points, achievable goals, clear outcomes, or measurable results.

Before you can set out to solve a problem in which the goals, outcomes, and results are unclear, you will need to attempt to transform a poorly defined problem into one that is well defined. How? By limiting the question statement. Difficult-to-define problems can range from those that are too vague--"What is the meaning of life?"--to those that further questioning can redefine and resolve--"Why is this patient unconscious?"

Narrow the focus of each part of the problem. In the vague "meaning of life" question, you will need to define the specific words--"meaning" and "life." Then you will need to identify the concrete, observable activities that fit your definition of "meaning" and "life." In the problem related to the patient, you will problem-solve through the steps of a differential diagnosis.

If you are baffled by a problem-solving question on an examination, ask yourself, "What is this question asking me to think about?" Perhaps you think that the exam question is poorly defined only because you cannot remember the relevant data. Under what conditions or circumstances will this problem be solvable? Break down the question into the component words and phrases and ask yourself questions about what you remember about the meaning of each word and phrase.

Problem-solving is closely related to logic and deductive reasoning. Whether or not you have classified yourself as a **Sensing** type, use your **Sensing** skills to take in all of the available data about the problem. Now use the specific **Intuitive, Thinking,** and **Feeling** rules of learning-style procedures.

Many hard-to-define problems are by nature so changeable, dynamic, and complicated that they foil even the best planned strategy. An apparently reasonable solution may seem unacceptable when more information is gathered, or when the circumstances of the poorly defined problem changes. In this case, simplify the language of the problem statement and limit the statement to a time and/or situation-specific context before you attempt to jump in and solve the problem.

In medicine, a well-defined problem may be one that asks you to intervene when a relatively healthy patient has a normal, garden-variety illness. You will need first to diagnose that the patient has a disease or condition; then to retrieve information about what the disease is, and what are the causes of the disease; and finally to determine what you can do to intervene. What steps--pharmacological, environmental, or surgical--must you take to reverse the disease process? Once you have a clear definition of the problem, you are ready for the next step.

An example of a difficult-to-define medical problem is one that poses the dilemma of value judgments. For example, what do you do when you are asked to choose between administering heroic medical intervention to an elderly, wealthy, famous dying patient, and providing expensive medical service to an indigent, uninsured younger patient with a good chance for recovery?

Problem-solving in this type of situation will ask you to refine and define the problem.

You will consider such issues as quality of life, ethical standards, legal constraints, cost-benefit realities, allocation of resources, research possibilities, family concerns, and probable outcome. As you consider these related issues, you will begin to formulate cause-effect subgoals.

DEVISE A STRATEGY--FORM SUBGOALS

The best way to refine the question statement of a problem is to limit it by forming subgoals. Whether the problem began as one that is well defined or ill defined, you will clarify the question by asking scientific, cause-effect questions: "If this, then what?"

A successful plan of attack requires you to divide the problem into logical steps that become the subgoals. As you conquer each subgoal, you will be able to reach the outcome asked for or implied by the problem statement.

In forming subgoals, look for underlying guiding principles. Use your logical, objective **Thinking** function to retrieve relevant information from the environment or from memory; sort out relevant from irrelevant information; derive or invent solution procedures for each subgoal; carry out these procedures logically, sequentially, efficiently, and correctly; verify your success at achieving both intermediate and terminal results.

To establish logical subgoals, you will need to:

1. reinterpret the problem description or statement

2. break down the problem into understandable steps or parts

3. follow rules, steps, or strategies, solving each subset as you go. These strategies can range from simplistic trial-and-error solutions, to more sophisticated scientific-method approaches, to reasoning by analogy

4. make assumptions and check them out by testing your hypothesis. Have you achieved each step in each of your subgoals?

5. move to the next step, following general rules or principles. In the event of failure to achieve subgoals, develop new assumptions as needed.

EXECUTE THE STRATEGY

Barring factors such as illness, fatigue, and momentary lapses in attention, executing the strategy is a straightforward process when you are working on simple, well defined problems. But when you are confronted with more complex problems, the problem-solving strategy will need to be comprehensive and well organized.

To plan an effective problem-solving strategy, you will need to ask if the problem is well defined. Now classify the *type* of problem that faces you, and determine the relative difficulty of the problem. What experiences have you had with problems of this type? Adhere to guiding principles. What is the problem analogous to? What are the consequences of each step of the solution? Use your **Thinking** skills to evaluate your strategies objectively. Stay focused on your goals, and narrow the possibilities of moves you will make.

If, for example, you wanted to determine which move to take in a game of chess, you would not start by considering all of the moves you could make. The number of possible moves is large, and the outcome of many of them is weak. Because you know the relative merits and shortcomings of the possible moves, a logical strategy would be to consider moving your powerful pieces first. The use of this strategy is based on your knowledge of the game and on your history of successes and failures in moving chess pieces.

In answering examination questions, your strategy is based on your knowledge of the rules "game" of the exam, on the subject content of the exam, and on your successes and failures in the past. Use your objective **Thinking** skills to evaluate how well you have broken down the problem into subgoals.

Workable strategies require a variety of skills. You need to *recall* specific information relevant to the problem. You may need to *apply* the information you know in a *new way*. You need to be inventive and flexible. You may draw a sketch, put the problem in other words, invent a model or representation. Often you must create analogies to understand the information referred to in the problem statement. If, for instance, the workings of the human eye baffle you, you will help yourself if you use an analogy representing the eye as a camera.

EVALUATE YOUR PROGRESS

Has the problem been solved? To know whether you are making progress toward the goal, you must decide whether you have enough information to carry out your current strategy, or whether you need to gather more information and devise a new strategy.

Go back to the first three steps in the learning-style problem-solving process-- **Sensing**, **Intuition**, and **Thinking**. Have you defined the problem accurately? Was your strategy an outgrowth of that definition? Were your subgoals appropriate to your definition? Did you use guiding principles to execute your initial strategy? Were you flexible, or did you base your strategy on erroneous and subjectively fixed assumptions?

Use your **Thinking** and **Feeling** --objective and subjective--dimensions to determine whether progress toward the goal has been achieved and whether the current strategy should be executed further or should be abandoned. If you decide objectively and subjectively that the present strategy is unworkable, then you will begin to redefine the problem, create new subgoals, and devise new strategies.

SUMMARY

As a physician-in-training, you have begun your lifelong professional problem- solving process through study, laboratory exercises, discussions, and test-taking. Examination success and your ability to retain the information you have learned is directly related to your ability to apply the steps of problem-solving techniques.

The steps in successful problem-solving are summarized as follows:

1. Know yourself and expand your learning style. Do not be limited by your learning-style preferences. Despite your personal preference for one or the other method of perceiving information and making decisions about it, be ready to use *all* mental functions--**Sensing**, **Intuition**, **Thinking**, and **Feeling**--one at a time and in order.

2. Define the problem. Be certain that you have understood the language of the problem. Transform an ill-defined problem into one that is well defined. Be able to determine the short-range and long-range goals.

3. Construct a strategy. Devise your strategy or plan of attack based on clear, achievable subgoals. Once more, proceed by using the mental functions in order--**Sensing**, **Intuition**, **Thinking**, **Feeling.** Use these mental functions within the energy contexts of **Extraversion**, then **Introversion.** Be sure that you use your **Perceiving** dimension to examine all the options, and your **Judging** attitude to stay on schedule.

4. Execute the strategy. Create models or analogies based on your recall of relevant information. Proceed from known information. Observe *what is*--**Sensing**--then develop a hypothesis of *what might be*--**Intuition**--and apply the old information in a new way. Objectively evaluate your progress as you proceed to execute the strategy. Follow objective, general principles of **Thinking**, and then use your **Feeling** function to determine subjectively if you are on the right track.

5. Evaluate your progress toward the goal. Did you solve the problem? Do you have enough information to execute your current strategy, or should you discard your strategy and devise a new one based on the rules and sequence of the problem-solving steps?

References

McCaulley, M. H. (1987) *Developing Critical Thinking and Problem-Solving Abilities: New Directions for Teaching and Learning.* San Francisco: Jossey-Bass, pp37-53

Scandura, J. M. (1977) *Problem Solving: A Structural/Process Approach with Instructional Implications.* New York: Academic Press

Wessells, M. G. (1982) *Cognitive Psychology.* New York: Harper and Row

Wilhite, S. C. (1990) Self-efficacy, locus of control, self-assessment of memory ability, and study activities as predictors of college course achievement *Journal of Educational Psychology* 82 (4) pp 696-700

Suggested Readings

Ackerman, P. L., Sternberg, R. J., and Glaser, R., Editors. (1989) *Learning and Individual Differences Advances in Theory and Research.* New York: W.H. Freeman and Co

Field, K., Cohler, B. J., Wool, G., Editors. (1989) *Learning and Education: Psychoanalytic Perspectives.*Madison, CT: International Universities Press, Inc

Kimble, D. P., Editor. (1967) *The Organization of Recall, Learning, Remembering, and Forgetting, Volume II,* The New York Academy of Sciences

Lehman, D. and Nisbett, R. (1990) A longitudinal study of the effects of undergraduate training on research. *Developmental Psychology* 26 (6) pp. 952-960

CHAPTER FIVE • PREPARING FOR NATIONAL BOARD EXAMINATIONS

Medical students faced with standardized tests often report that they know more than they are able to demonstrate on an examination. Under the pressure of an exam, students may choose answers that are a product of guessing rather than of certainty or confidence in decision-making. Lack of confidence is often the result of inadequate or unsystematic preparation. To build confidence while preparing for an examination, you need to identify your strengths and weaknesses, know the exam format, know the subjects, know how to integrate the material, and know how to solve problems.

Purpose

This chapter will provide you with a system of comprehensive, time-efficient review strategies for the National Board of Medical Examiners Part I Examination. On completion of the exercises in this chapter, you will be able to:

- know the focus of the examination
- plan and apply strategies for a time-efficient and comprehensive review
- identify your academic strengths and weaknesses
- develop and use a comprehensive Organ System/Pathology Review integrating the biomedical sciences learned in the first two years of medical school
- increase your recall and reasoning abilities during study and test-taking
- increase your confidence in answer selection during examinations
- improve your test scores

MIND YOUR MIND

Guard against boredom as you review for the Boards. Unlike the starry-eyed freshman you once were, you no longer feel the rush of excitement at the novelty of the material. Jaded and sophisticated, you may be disappointed that you cannot approach the material with the initial buzz you experienced when you first met the stuff. The honeymoon is over! But as in all lasting relationships, affection can increase if we face reality and accept the mundane. Full understanding and knowledge can grow deeper with persistence, routine, and practice (Shain and Kelliher, 1988).

THE EXAM

In order to know what and how to study, you need information about the content, format, and scope of the NBME examination. According to the information released in *The National Board Examiner*, Part I of the National Boards is designed "to determine if an examinee understands and can apply key concepts of basic biomedical science, with an emphasis on principles and mechanisms of health, disease, and modes of therapy" (Anderson, 1990).

The Board tells us that the examination "will be constructed from an integrated content outline that organizes basic science material along three dimensions . . .
- organizational level (e.g., molecular, cellular, organ, whole person)
- process (different types of normal and abnormal processes)
- system (e.g., cardiovascular, musculoskeletal, reproductive)."

This exam focus and form will demand corresponding study strategies as you prepare to show what you know. In the construction of questions, four important differences have been instituted in the NBME examinations commencing with June 1991.

These are:
- a decrease in the percentage of items requiring recall of isolated facts
- an increase in the percentage requiring comprehension and reasoning

• a predominance of the questions that ask for one-best-answer (A-type)

    and matching (B-type) items

• the absence of multiple true/false (K-type) and

    A/B/Both/Neither (C-type) items

REVIEW STRATEGIES

From the first day you decided to attend medical school, you began to prepare for the National Medical Board Examination. You studied biomedical science because you were interested in putting theory into practice. The NBME--a summary of your efforts--is the next step along the path toward the practice of medicine.

As you face the prospect of the exam head-on, you may wish you had more time to prepare. Perhaps you feel that you didn't learn enough. But once you start to put it all together, you will be happy to find that you know more than you think you do. In the time you have set aside to review and integrate your studies, you will need to organize, analyze, and synthesize your knowledge. Let's put together a plan of action.

Plan

A good carpenter takes time to sharpen the saw before beginning the building process. Time and study focus are your tools. Therefore, you will want to plan your attack:

• Allow adequate *time* for review of subjects and organ systems.

• Develop strategies for *time* conservation.

• Take *time* to develop a workable schedule, and organize your personal life with

    attention to maximum energy efficiency.

• Attend to your physical and psychological well-being during the period of *time*

    in which you prepare for and take the examination.

Subject Coverage

Students who are overwhelmed by the review process report that when they begin to study, they feel as though they have forgotten everything they ever knew. In order to quell their anxiety, fearful students tend to make the mistake of going over and over material they know. Spending time this way wastes the opportunity to tackle problem subjects.

Anxiety-avoiding students may not be conscious of the fact that they are afraid to face their weak areas. You must attend to all the material, spending more time on those subjects that gave you trouble, less time on your strong subjects.

Appreciate your strengths, and close gaps in your knowledge. To organize the task ahead, before tackling review books, spend about 20 hours looking through *everything*: course outlines and syllabi, tables of contents in texts, and your own class notes. Pay particular attention to your labels and underlining. In scanning the whole terrain, you will become aware of how much you remember and where your areas of concern may be. Once you have gone through everything, use the Oklahoma Notes to take pretests, making an objective determination of your strengths and weaknesses.

Divide your answers into three categories:

1. "know it cold" +++
2. "not too sure" +- ?
3. "don't know"   - -?

Time Use

Once you have determined the extent of your knowledge, you will want to schedule at least two thirds of your allotted time on the "not too sure" and "don't know" areas. If you have two months for exam preparation, obviously you won't have time for a thorough review of every word of two years' notes, texts, references, and laboratory findings. Unlike classroom exams, in which you use a cram-it-all-in-before-the-test method, your review strategy for the National Boards will mandate a selective study approach. Weak areas get more time.

Use an appointment book and a large wall-chart in full view of your desk to tabulate the time you spend on each subject and on each organ system. Keep tabs of the time you work alone and with your study group. By now you know how long you can sit still at your desk. Schedule breaks. Schedule small oases of time to phone or to be with energy-restoring family and friends.

Set Priorities--Scheduling

Set up a structured time schedule for reviewing each area. Work at the same time each day. When you set your schedule, pay attention to your energy highs and lows. At what time of day do you feel full of vim? When are you drooping? Remember to save high-energy times for the subjects that give you difficulty, and low-energy times for easier, better known material.

Plan the days that you will spend on each subject area. Intersperse short sessions of your favorites among the long bouts with the tough areas. Use the Tricks and Treats method discussed in Chapter Two • Time Management and Memory.

Retake the tests in the Oklahoma Notes after you have reviewed a topic. In addition to giving you practice in answering Board-type questions, this pretest, posttest method will increase your motivation and sustain concentration as you pace yourself through the time you have allotted for review.

Keep a record of the areas you have mastered. As you work, subject by subject, through the review books, use the chart above your desk to enter a visual reminder of the material you have covered. In an appointment book, make note of the pages you have read, review books gone through, and test scores achieved. When you feel bogged down, you will be able to look at your chart and your appointment book and feel confident as you celebrate your progress at confronting your weak areas.

Once you have overcome deficiencies in your weakest subject areas, then your task will be learning, clarifying, and reviewing your material with an eye to integration. Save time during the last three weeks prior to the exam to pull the subjects together in an organ system/pathology review.

INTEGRATING SUBJECTS: ORGAN SYSTEM/PATHOLOGY REVIEW

The questions on National Boards are comprehensive and interdisciplinary, so in addition to testing yourself with the more simple subject-by-subject review method presented in the Oklahoma Notes, you will want to use a more complex method of study integration provided by an organ system/pathology review.

Remember that your goal is to prepare and study along the lines of the exam format "with an emphasis on principles and mechanisms of health, disease, and modes of therapy" (NBME, 1990).

The organ system/pathology strategy is not only an invaluable organizing method for a comprehensive review but also useful preparation for clinical work. This mode of study integrates and applies the important relationships between an organ structure, its function, its mechanism of action; the differences between normal and abnormal conditions; and the diseases and pathological conditions affecting each organ system.

Setting Up an Organ System/Pathology Review

To my knowledge, there are no specific Board Review books that spell out an integrative system for a review based on an organ system or pathology method. Even if such a book did exist, it would not be as relevant as the system we will construct in this chapter. You are about to become the author of your own personal review book.
Let's begin.

In order to master the areas you feel weak in, pick an organ system that you felt unsure of when you studied it for the first time. Is that system renal, cardiac, respiratory, adrenal, other? Identify the organ system in the space below.

Target Organ System_____

Once you have chosen the specific organ system, together we will develop a question matrix for it. As you systematically apply a question matrix to your weakest area of knowledge, we will proceed to apply the matrices to all the other organ systems. You will be pleasantly surprised at how much you actually do remember.

FOUR-STEP STRATEGY

Question Matrix Steps

The following organ system four-step strategy (Schwenker, 1987) will allow you to create a question matrix based on a well-organized, comprehensive, systematic format.

1. Build a question matrix beginning with the gross anatomy of the organ--its structure. Identify all parts, relationships, size, shape, appearance, and every aspect of the *structure*. Next, include the *embryogenesis*, then the changes that occur with *development* and *maturation*. Now add *histological structure*, and the *characteristics* of the *cells* and *cell types* that constitute the organ. Be sure your matrix includes *details* and *concepts*. Remember that the "What is . . .?" questions test your recall, and the *concepts* questions--"What patterns" and "What would happen if . . .?"--test your application of information and deductive reasoning abilities.

2. Identify the *physiological* and *biochemical processes* extant in the organ. Note the chemicals the organ *secretes*; the *biochemical synthesis* of the compounds and how they are *degraded*; the *relationships* between the *histological*, *cellular*, *biochemical*, and *physiological functions*. What will you expect to find in *normal functioning*?

3. Move toward pathology by identifying the *results* in terms of *cause* and *effect* of the *biochemical* and *physiological processes* that are in operation owing to *excesses* or *deficiencies* in hormones, vitamins, minerals, secretions . . . . What are the different *types of pathology* that might affect the organ? What *abnormalities* might you expect to find? What are the organ's *responses to the pathologic processes*?, e.g., infectious organisms, neoplasms, toxic reactions, inflammation. What occurs in the organ and in

other organ systems when the organ attempts to repair itself?

4. Identify the *types of pharmacological* and *clinical interventions* that would directly affect the *structure, function,* and *mechanism of action* of the physiology and biochemistry of the organ? What medications or groups of drugs are used in the event of disease or illness? What groups of drugs or medications will *modify the effects* of the compounds produced by the organ?

While you are creating the four-step method, notice the *labels*, which are emphasized by *special print* The labels should be in your notes, ready for you to pull out and use for question construction. When you find these labels in your notes, you are ready to construct a sample question matrix.

If you are still not too sure about how to plunge in with your own question matrix, let's try a question matrix exercise, applying the four-step method to the renal system. Once you have completed this exercise, you will develop your own matrix related to the organ system that caused you difficulty when you first studied it.

For purposes of emphasis, specific identifying words that appeared in your notes as *labels* are here in *italics*. The italicized words are usually the pivotal words found in comprehensive examination questions. They are the words that tell you what the question is about. Learn to see them. As you move through the exercise, answer the questions and add any other questions that occur to you.

118

Renal System Organ System Review

Where is the kidney *located* in *relation* to other *structures*?

What are the *parts* of the *structure* of the kidney?

Draw the *structures* in the space below.

What specific *function* does each *part* of the kidney perform?

What is the *derivation* of the blood supply?

What are the *origins* and *pathways* of the nerve supply? What *types* of nerves are found: sensory? motor?

Describe and diagram the *steps* of the following processes. Indicate the *requirements*, and *results* in terms of *cause* and *effect*, of each step of each process.

1. Filtration:

2. Reabsorption:

3. Secretion:

4. Excretion:

Name the *parts* of the nephron. What *function* does each part perform?

Consider *embryogenesis* and *development*. What cells are the embryological *precursors* of the *parts* of the kidney?

Consider the renal system *developmentally*: What *changes* does the kidney undergo?

What does the kidney *do*?

By what *mechanism of action* does the kidney perform its *function*?

Create diagrams that show the *mechanisms of action*.

How are the kidney's compounds *formed biochemically*?

What are the *physiological effects* of the hormone secretions of the organ?

What are the *results* of each *function* of the kidney in terms of *cause and effect*?

What are the *products* of degradation?

Name and draw the *steps* in the normal physiological *mechanisms* and *range* of *normal* activity?

What are the most *common diseases* and *pathological states* occurring in the kidney?

How do these abnormal states *present clinically*?

What *laboratory studies* might you seek in the event of the above illnesses?

What are the *normal laboratory findings*?

What are the disease *incidences, demographics, age, race,* and any *environmental risks* or *exogenous factors* that may impact on the renal system?

In the disease process, how do *bacteria, viruses,* and *parasites* affect the kidney?

What *kinds of tumors* will occur in the kidney, and what are their *effects*?

What are the possible *effects of surgery* on the renal system?

What happens when one kidney is *removed*?

Describe the *external mechanical system* designed to perform the functions of the kidney?

How does dialysis work? What are the *indications* for and *risk factors* in the use of dialysis?

What are the *indications* and *contraindications* for, the *risks*, and the *effects* of a kidney transplant?

What can be done to *intervene pharmacologically* to avoid kidney surgery, or to *reverse* the *disease states* of the kidney?

What *other disease states* in the body affect the kidney?

How do you *test* for diseases and/or illnesses that affect the kidney?

What are the possible *iatrogenic results* to the kidney caused by the treatment of other illnesses?

What are the *histological* and *functional effects* of long-term steroid therapy?

What are the *histological* and *functional effects* of kidney disease caused by long-term diabetes mellitus?

How does a *normal condition* like pregnancy affect the kidney? Why?

How might *other conditions* in the body and the administration of certain medications affect the organ?

How do you *prevent* diseases of the renal system?

Create diagrams and describe the renal system and its *relationship* to other *organs* and *organ systems*.

Add questions related to *immunology, virology, parasitology*, or any other subject areas that occur to you as you go through your review.

Once you have reviewed the components of this question matrix, please choose an organ system that gave you difficulty when you were studying it for the first time. Using the renal system question matrix as your guide, construct, on a separate sheet of paper, your own organ system question matrix. Remember to keep in mind the italicized labels from your notes as you go through your exercise.

Target Organ System_____

Use of Study Partners in the Comprehensive Review

During the frenzy of attempting to cover the entire first two years in just two months, most students elect to study alone. This is a mistake. Although studying alone may give you the illusion of covering a great deal of material in a short amount of time, solitary study will allow your knowledge gaps to go unnoticed.

You will find that you can plug your knowledge holes, and cut your work time in half, if you study with a reliable study partner. Keeping in mind that the best way to learn is to teach, you will be forced to put into words what you know and make known those areas you may not feel too certain about. Do not use your study partner to show off what you know. Spend your time only in working through your "not too sure" and "don't know" subject areas.

Prepare for your study-partner sessions as you would for a classroom recitation session. First work alone, using personally constructed question matrices that cover your areas of weakness. Then work twice weekly with a study partner, in sessions lasting about two hours each. Together you will start with the subject-by-subject review method, then later you will add the organ system review.

Your study partner should be unlike you in learning style. So if you are a **Sensor**-- liking details, being present-oriented, and preferring to study in a sequential organization--find an **Intuitive** as your complementary partner. The **Intuitive** will prefer to focus on concepts, will be future-oriented, and will help you by asking "What would happen if . . .?" questions.

Intuitive learning-style partners find tangential information exciting; therefore, you will be encouraged to make associations while you study. Of course, the **Intuitive** will benefit by the here-and-now practicality of the **Sensor's** study techniques.

This buddy system will take advantage of all of the mental functions you use to take in information--**Sensing**, **Intuition**, **Thinking**, and **Feeling** (McCaulley, 1987). As you review, you will utilize the *details* you have amassed by using your **Sensing** skills in the subject-by-subject method. You will reinforce the *concepts* you studied and developed through the use of your **Intuitive** skills. You will ask yourself to use your **Thinking** skills and be objective as you answer the questions. Then you will question yourself, "Does this **Feel** right to me subjectively?"

Sensors prefer to follow a plan of subject-by-subject review. **Intuitives** are intrigued and stimulated by the complexities of an organ system/pathology review. No matter what your learning style, you will need to do both.

The subject-by-subject review will assure that you have covered all of the facts you need to recall. The comprehensive organ system/pathology review method will enable you to integrate the basic biomedical science subjects you have learned in your preclinical years.

Once you have worked through both the subject-by-subject and the organ system review, alone and with your study partner, you will find that you will save much time and cut down on knowledge-gap frustration if you work for at least two hours weekly in a larger, more dynamic study environment--the study group. See Chapter Eight • Organizing and Working In A Study Group for specific tips on time-efficient, comprehensive methods to complete your review by working in groups.

SUMMARY

Time and study focus are the main concerns during your review process. Use a pretest, posttest system to determine what you know and don't know. Adhere to a schedule. You will use at least two thirds of your exam preparation time on your weakest areas. Study each separate subject first, then put the subjects together in a comprehensive organ system/pathology review.

Use an opposite learning-style-type study partner to help you clarify the fuzzy areas, discuss the material you have mastered, and deepen your understanding. In the last four weeks of review, spend at least two hours weekly with a study partner and two hours weekly in a study group comprising different learning-style types. Use the mental functions in order: **Sensing**, **Intuition**, **Thinking**, and **Feeling**.

Develop your organ system/pathology review by identifying the organ system that you know least about, and then use a four-step question matrix:

1. Begin with the gross anatomy of the organ. Include the embryogenesis, changes that occur with development and maturation, histological structure, and the characteristics of the cells and cell types that constitute the organ.

2. Identify the physiological and biochemical processes extant in the organ: the chemicals the organ secretes; the biochemical synthesis of the compounds and how they are degraded; the relationships between the histological, cellular, biochemical, and physiological functions. Be sure you know normal values.

3. Consider the pathology that might develop in the organ. What abnormalities might you expect to find? What are the organ responses to the pathologic processes?

4. Identify the types of pharmacological and clinical interventions that would directly affect the structure, function, mechanism of action, and physiologic and biochemical processes of the organ? What medications or groups of drugs would modify the effects of the compounds produced by the organ?

You have done all that you can do to prepare for your exams. You can now proceed with confidence. If you feel shaky and under stress, let's take care of that stress now by going through the exercises in the next chapter, Stress Management.

References

Anderson, R. E., M.D., Chairman for the Comprehensive Part I Examination, et al. *The National Board Examiner* Vol 37, No 1. Winter 1990 Philadelphia, PA, National Board of Medical Examiners, Pub.

McCaulley, M. H. (1987) *Developing Critical Thinking and Problem-Solving Abilities: New Directions for Teaching and Learning,* San Francisco, CA: Jossey-Bass

Schwenker, J. A. (1987) *Student Information Manual.* Medical College of Wisconsin: Office of Academic Affairs

Shain, D. D. and Kelliher, G. J. (1988) A study skills workshop as an integral part of orientation to medical school: The establishment of self-directed learning. *Proceedings of the Twenty-Seventh Annual Conference Research in Medical Education* Chicago, Illinois. Assoc. of Amer. Medical Colleges pp 91-96

CHAPTER SIX · STRESS MANAGEMENT

Pre-exam tension interferes with your ability to remember, concentrate, and think clearly. Fear of failure or, for some people, the fear of success can create tension and stress. When your education process requires the rapid acquisition of too much new information with not enough time for understanding and integration, unhealthy stress can result. While studying and while taking exams, if you can take control, recognize, manage, and eliminate stress, you will increase your possibilities for pleasure, learn more, and improve your examination scores (Carver and Scheier, 1982; Perry and Penner, 1990; Rothbaum, Weisz, and Snyder, 1982).

Purpose

The purpose of this chapter is to enable you to recognize the early warning signs of tension and stress, and to take immediate steps to combat the transitory stress that occurs during study sessions and while taking exams. This chapter is not a comprehensive study of stress, nor will it attempt to address all of the causes and effects of stress. In some instances, stress is so overwhelming that return to a productive study focus and optimal performance on exams is possible only with psychotherapy.

CAUSES OF TRANSITORY STRESS

Engaging in any activity that implies evaluation can result in performance anxiety. Unrealistic expectations and too much to learn with not enough time to learn it can damage your ability to integrate all that you must master. Shifting from old, comfortably familiar ideas to rapid new knowledge acquisition can leave you feeling overloaded or, at times, immobilized. Discomfort and stress are compounded when you know that rapidly acquired, new, and troublesome material will be the very stuff that is sure to appear on the next exam. When you are stressed, exams seem to conspire to catch you at your worst.

The constant shift from feelings of competence to feeling like a dolt tips the scales of emotional stability for any learner under pressure. Worry about the possibility that you may not do well can, if left unattended, damage your self-esteem and compromise your performance. Negative emotions can range from mild discomfort to more severe and debilitating feelings of fear, shame, rejection, helplessness, and hopelessness. Discomfort must be attended to. Unattended discomfort can produce chronic, performance-compromising stress. The first step in reversing this stress is to regain a belief in your ability to take control of yourself and your study regimen.

SELF-EFFICACY

Educational self-efficacy is defined as "the extent to which students believe that they can control the outcomes of their attempts at learning" (Wilhite, 1990). Significant research was conducted to examine the possible relationships between student study behaviors and academic achievement (Christopoulus, Rohwer, and Thomas, 1987). Self-efficacy, locus of control, self-assessment of memory ability, and study activities were considered as they relate to examination succes. (Wilhite, 1990). These studies found that the single best predictor of achievement was the presence of a measure of self-efficacy.

The presence of self-efficacy reduces stress. Belief in yourself and your power to succeed is evident in encouraging internal dialogues that you sustain with yourself during times of academic challenge. Take a moment to hear your "self talk" when you study and when you take exams.

Are your messages to yourself negative or positive? If you tell yourself you are a failure, you will be. If you tell yourself you *can* do well, you *will* do well. Remember the fable of your childhood, "The Little Engine That Could"? *You* are that engine! You can succeed if you too will say, "I think I can, I think I can . . . . "

SIGNS OF STRESS

When you are under extreme stress, your body copes in ways that are obvious to you and to others. Your pulse races, your mouth becomes dry, your digestive system goes haywire, your hands perspire, your sexual interest wanes, and your muscles tense. Many times, however, the stress response is more subtle and less consciously noticeable. When you are in this less obvious stressed condition, your circulatory system responds, your sense of well-being is compromised, and your capacity for learning is diminished.

Stress reactions often lead to harmful habits. They can include excesses of drinking, eating, smoking, and drug use. Your body often responds to unattended stress with headaches, back pain, loss of energy, insomnia, or hypersomnia. When you least expect to lose control, you may find yourself shouting or snapping at friends.

STRESS REDUCTION TECHNIQUES

Unless the stress is symptomatic of unresolved conflicts or serious emotional problems, replacing your negative thoughts with positive action strategies can often combat stress. Psychologists tell us that positive results can be achieved if you move from feeling like a victim taking charge of your destiny (Seligman, 1975). You can mobilize stress and make discomfort a force for success if you identify stressors and evaluate the reality of the stressful situation. When you are aware that you are stressed, there are steps you can take to regain your composure and self-confidence.

The stress you feel as an overworked, sleep-deprived medical student can derive from your belief that you simply cannot afford the time to take a break. Nonsense! You can't afford not to! Although you may think that taking a break requires time you simply don't have, there are many quick and easy stress reduction techniques you can use.

Students under pressure find that stress reduction is possible through brief interludes of prayer, meditation, deep-breathing exercises, and yoga (Shain and Kelliher, 1988). If you already have a method that works for you, use it. The following supplementary exercises can be added to yours. They can be done while studying, before going to sleep, and during exams.

Developing Positive Self-Talk

Do you like yourself? Do you treat yourself with respect? Are you generous with yourself? When you take time to relax, do you tell yourself that you deserve to take a guilt-free break? Do you celebrate the fact that you are talented enough to be in medical school? Do you know that if you work through each subject day by day, and step by step, you will probably know enough to pass your exams? Can you remember a time when you felt happy with yourself? What were you doing that felt good? Were you helping someone else? Now be the caring person you were then, and learn to care for yourself.

Eliminating Negative Self-Talk

Do you worry about not succeeding? Do you feel that you are an impostor, giving colleagues, friends, family, and instructors false impressions of your competence? Do you secretly believe that you are not worthy of the right to practice medicine? Do you fear evaluation, believing that your past successes have been due to luck or error?

Do you worry that if you *do* succeed you will be rejected by your family or be cast out of your circle of nonmedical friends? Recognize what you are doing and stop this negative cycle now! It will do you in. If, after completing the following exercises, you can't seem to stop the negative self-talk, then get professional help.

Exercises for Identifying and Improving Self-Talk

In seeking personal and professional success, the words you say to yourself can be either stumbling blocks or your keys to the kingdom. In the space below, please write your impression of yourself as a potential success or failure as a practicing physician.

Why will I make a good doctor?

What can I tell myself if someone implies that I am incompetent?

If I truly *am* incompetent, what can I do to develop competence?

What words will it take for me to change a negative statement to a positive message about myself?

Take a moment to think about your past academic record. You didn't always feel worried about yourself, did you? Could a temporary crisis of confidence have occurred when you demanded too much of yourself?

In order to remind yourself that you deserve to be in medical school, name, in the space below, all your past academic successes. If you need more space, gather extra paper and celebrate yourself.

Evaluating Your Attitude Toward Examinations

Perhaps you feel that you will be a fine doc but worry that you will not be able to jump the academic hurdles you will need to negotiate to get there. Maybe you don't do as well on examinations as you should. You know more than the paper says you do. This know-more, do-less phenomenon may be due to stress factors and your attitude before, during, and after examinations.

To tune in to your emotional state when you take examinations, please complete the following sentences:

When I study for examinations, I usually feel . . .

When I take an examination, I usually tell myself that I . . .

During the exam, I usually feel . . .

Immediately after the exam, I usually feel . . .

When I get the results of my exam, I usually feel . . .

Look at the messages you have written above. During all the stages of preparation, taking the test, and aftertest review, do you feel mostly confident or mostly anxious?

Imagine yourself as you would like to feel while studying each day's work. Please write that scenario in the space below.

Because everyone fears the worst-case scenario--failure--let's imagine several stages in that eventuality.

What would happen if:

•you were called on during a recitation session and you had no idea about the answer?

• you barely passed an exam?

• you failed the next exam?

• you failed a course?

• you failed a whole semester?

• you passed everything but could not pass the National Board Examinations?

• you failed everything so badly that you would have to consider another profession?

Are any of these horror statements life-threatening? Probably not, but life-threatening is how most success-oriented people view the possibility of failure. Failure can be viewed as an end to the possibility of a meaningful life, or it can be an opportunity to determine what you need to do next time so that you will succeed.

Negative scripts etch themselves into the psyche. Failure-fear creates stress and drains the psyche of energy. So what a failure-worrier worries about, he actually brings about!

DEMONSTRATION OF NEGATIVE OR POSITIVE THINKING

When introduced to many people at a party, you have heard people say, "I never remember names." And indeed they don't! Could it be because they have programmed themselves to forget? Might they be attempting to absolve themselves from the responsibility to remember? Negative self-statements stick.

Try this experiment if you want to see the result of negative self-talk on your energy.

Stand upright with your back to a friend or colleague. Extend your arms out from your shoulders like this:

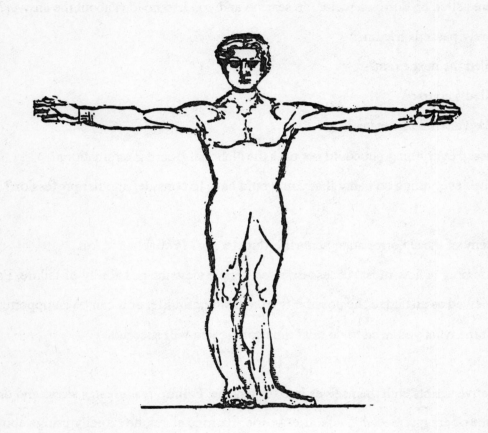

Have a friend stand behind you. Think of as many positive statements about yourself as you can. Now say those positive statements aloud. Proclaim with a voice of conviction that you are bright, capable, witty, and will be able to accomplish anything you set your mind on. Search your mind and find any other positive things about yourself that you truly believe, and say them aloud. While you do this, keep your arms extended from the shoulder. Ask your friend to attempt to pull your dominant arm down to your side while you do your best to resist the pull.

Now stand in the same position. This time think of negative things about yourself. Say aloud anything you don't like about yourself. Say that you are a failure, a fraud, will probably hate the practice of medicine, and any other negative appraisal that has ever been heaped on you. Once more, as before, keep your arms extended from your shoulders and have your friend attempt to pull your dominant arm to your side while you fight to resist the pull.

If you are like the hundreds of other students I have worked with who have completed this exercise, you will discover that when you provide yourself with positive self-talk, you have the energy to resist being pulled down, whereas if you have a tendency to attribute negative characteristics to yourself, you will not have the energy to resist a downward force. Your ability to remain upright and stable is directly affected by what you say to yourself about yourself.

Get the message? From now on, if you want to develop your talents, positive self-talk is all you will permit yourself while you study and while you demonstrate the results of your study efforts during exams.

Give yourself a pep talk. See yourself possessing the knowledge you want to have. Feel your competence in your bones. If there is something you don't know now, be challenged by it, confident that eventually you will learn it.

Enjoy yourself as you take measures to find the answers you want. Your patients and you will benefit from your optimism, curiosity, and compassion. Remember that compassion for your patients begins with compassion for yourself.

STRESS-REDUCTION EXERCISES

The Alexander Technique

In 1892, F.M. Alexander, a Shakespearean actor, discovered a significant relationship between the alignment of a person's head, neck, and back during times of relaxation and during stress. When Alexander became anxious during a performance, his body responded with tension, thereby causing him to be hoarse and lose his voice. Alexander was curious about why this happened. Could it be that his tension led to the problem?

Alexander discovered--after many years of kinesiology and anatomy research-- that with tension, a person's head leaves its optimal upright angle. This shifting of the balance of the head and neck results in an out-of-alignment position, adding physical tension to an already emotionally tense body. The resulting tension can be felt in the trapezius, sternocleidomastoid, occipital triangle, and supraclavicular triangle muscles.

In 1926, the physiologist Rudolf Magnus of Utrecht discussed the physiology of posture. Magnus pointed out that the optimal mechanism of the body acts in such a way that the head leads and the body follows.

Students engaged in long study sessions variously assume two characteristic positions. In one, the chin juts forward, the head is pulled back, and the muscles at the back of the neck shorten; in the other, the head falls forward from the seventh cervical, the shoulders round, and the muscles of the chest are drawn together. In either position, tension abounds.

You can relieve that tension by observing and correcting the positions you use. The tension-producing and the optimal positions of the head and neck, and consequent body alignment, are illustrated on the page that follows (Westfeldt, 1964).

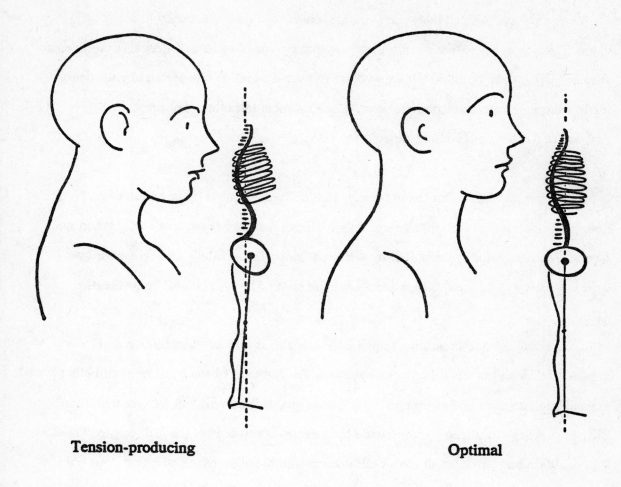

Tension-producing   Optimal

While you are engaged in long periods of sedentary activity, such as studying and taking examinations, protect your body from tension. Allow your body to work at its peak efficiency by mentally directing your head to move up and away from your shoulders.

This mental process of *permitting* freedom from tension will allow your head to move upward in space from an imaginary point on the sagittal suture, just behind the coronal suture. As you work at your desk, take the time to pay attention to your head, neck, and back alignment. Do not add undue physical stressors that create unnecessary exhaustion and tension. To get the full benefit of optimal head, neck, and body alignment, add gentle deep-breathing exercises to your body-alignment regimen.

Breathing

You may have noticed that when you are tense, you have a tendency to sigh or to yawn. This is your body's way of telling you that you need fuller and deeper air intake and output. A few deep breaths will help you to release tension. While seated at your desk, while studying, or even during an exam, take a moment to notice your breathing. Are you utilizing your full lung capacity?

If you want to know how to breathe, watch a sleeping baby, lying on his back. Notice how his belly rises with air intake and falls with exhalation. Maybe that's why when we awake after a refreshing sleep, we say we have "slept like a baby." Observe your own breathing just as you are falling asleep. Like the relaxed baby, you will belly-breathe.

To practice relaxed breathing, here are the steps to assure a full inhalation and exhalation: Place your hand on your abdomen. As you take a breath, allow your belly to expand so that your hand moves out with the air intake. You will feel fat, like a balloon filling up. Allow the air to remain inside for a second or two. Feel the full feeling. Then, as if the balloon has burst, let all the air out with an audible sigh. Make sure that your body expels *all* of the air. Repeat this procedure for at least three breaths.

Use this exercise in class, while studying, and before going to sleep. If you feel tense or tired during study sessions or during exams, be sure to take the time to revive yourself with a refreshing breath, attending to both inhalation and exhalation. Add a visual representation to your deep breathing.

Sit comfortably in a relaxed position, the top of your head lifting skyward. Close your eyes. Concentrate on breathing in through your nose and out through your mouth. Take gentle, slow, complete breaths. Each time you inhale, picture the word "RELAX" painted on your closed eyelids. As you continue the slow, rhythmic breathing, visualize yourself relaxing under a tropical sun on the smooth white sand of a quiet beach. You are soothed by the sun and the sounds of the sea and the distant undulating gulls. Breath all of this in as you feel yourself relaxing. Now let your exhalation mingle with the sea breeze in your mind.

Physical Exercise

We all have learned the value of exercise as part of a stress reduction plan. To reduce stressful muscle tension, make sure that you engage in an exercise routine that involves deep breathing and stretching . Walking, running, swimming, dancing, yoga, or any other activity that involves your large muscles will revive and preserve energy. Promise yourself a daily period of exercise. In the space below, write that promise. What activity will you use? When?

What_____When_____

Before you get ready to go to sleep at night, or when shifting from studying one subject to another, incorporate full body stretches with your study routine. Suppose that you have read 60 pages of a subject and you are ready to put that book aside and begin another task. It's time to attend to your body.

Punctuate study sessions with five minutes of stretching exercises. Lie on your back, arms extended from your shoulders so that your body forms a cross. Bend your knees, keeping your feet flat to the floor. Now bring your knees to your chest. Take in a full breath. As you gently release the air with a slow exhalation, let your knees drop slowly to one side. Return your knees to your chest, take in a full abdominal breath, allow your knees to fall to the other side while releasing the breath with a complete exhalation.

Repeat the procedure as you move from side to side two more times.

Spot-Check Mini-Exercises to be Done During Studying and Exams

You will be surprised how fast tension in the facial muscles can create exhaustion. Put your second and third digits together as one unit. Audibly tap your fingers on your forehead between your eyebrows. Is your brow furrowed? Do you detect tension? When you begin the tapping, do you notice a release of tension and a widening of the space between your eyebrows?

Tap again, as if you were attempting to percuss a patient's back or chest. While you tap, drop your jaw as if you were about to fall asleep. Imagine your face getting wider and longer as you let all tension go from your temporalis, masseter, occipitofrontalis, corrugator supercilii, sternocleidomastoid, procerus, medial, and lateral pterygoid muscles. (How's that for a review of the facial muscles?)

Now let's move down from your face. Notice the presence of any tension in your neck and between your shoulders? Slowly turn your chin first to one shoulder then to the other. Allow your head to move as far as it will go so that your chin touches first one and then the other shoulder. Now bend your from head side to side as you touch your ear, first to one shoulder, then to the other.

To give your upper limb, shoulder, and back muscles a full stretch, grasp your hands behind your back behind your chair. Pull your hands down toward the floor so that your shoulders leave their tense and elevated position and move down from your ears.

By now you have used a few seconds to identify and release physical tension from your face, neck, and shoulders. You are ready to return to work with renewed energy and vigor. But what if you recognize that the tension is not only physical, that there is a negative mental spiral occurring? It's important that you take the time to replace those stressful negative images with ones that are positive.

Restful Images

Two thoughts cannot reside in your mind at the same time. So when tension begins to mount during a study session or in the midst of an exam, you can release the tension with a quick visit to a restful place. How do you do that? In your mind's eye!

Think of your favorite place. Imagine the most peaceful landscape you have ever seen. How does it look? What colors, sounds, and smells abound there? Make sure the spot is entirely neutral and pleasant. Don't pick a spot that is emotionally laden or is alive with memories. Conjure up any pleasant place in or out of this world.

If you can't think of any spot of your own, try thinking about any of these: a welcoming gentle brook, a supple tree swaying in a warm breeze, butter melting on a plate placed on a sunny windowsill. Once you have the image in mind, imagine that you can paint it on the inside of your eyelids. Write a description of your place of refuge in the space below:

Now calmly look up to the ceiling, the way you would if you were trying to remember a forgotten phone number. Let your eyelids drop gently over your uplifted eyes. Visualize your refuge setting; notice the colors; hear the sounds; take in the smells.

Move your eyes from right to left and from top to bottom of the scene. Take in a full, belly-expanding breath. Let the scene enter your whole body. After a five- to ten-second visit, open your eyes and return to your study or exam-taking tasks. Imaginary mini-vacations leave you refreshed and ready to do your best work.

Involving Your Family and Friends

Long periods of solitary work and study can be lonely. The best antidote to the toxic stress of isolation is the promise of fun. Take momentary breaks in your study routine to contact a loved one by telephone. Limit the length of the call so you do not consume too much valuable time. Tell that special someone how you feel about the pressure you are under and what you plan to do to relax. Try to find your sense of humor as you describe your endeavors.

Expect them to be interested as you tell them what you are studying. Explain the details and concepts that are the focus of your current study efforts. Let your trusted pal know what the next exam will cover and how soon it will be before you can take time out to "play" again. Set up an appointment for a well-deserved respite. The promise of a break might be all it takes to rejuvenate a flagging mind.

Now, physician-in-training, you have the tools you need to recognize and to combat stress. You can use them whenever you want, and in whatever setting. A burned-out student makes an inefficient scholar.

A stressed-out doctor makes an inefficient diagnostician. "Physician, heal thyself!"

SUMMARY

The pressures of time and performance anxiety, by definition, lead to stress. Stress leads to self-defeating inefficiency and poor judgment. You need not become an unwilling victim of stress. You can take action. Take charge. Give yourself a dose of optimism and positive self-talk. Take time to add stress reduction exercises to your study regimen. Allow yourself to admit that there is no such thing as personal or professional perfection. We are all works in progress. You are in medical school because you are bright and competent and you want to help other people. Start by helping yourself.

References

Carver, C.S. and Scheier, M.F. (1982) Control theory: A useful conceptual framework for personality-social, clinical, and health psychology. *Psychological Bulletin,* 92. pp 111-135

Christopoulos, J.P., Rohwer, W.D., Jr., and Thomas, J.W. (1987) Grade level differences in students' study activities as a function of course characteristics. *Contemporary Educational Psychology,* 12, 303-323

Perry, R.P. and Penner, K.S. (1990) Enhancing academic achievement in college students through attributional retraining and instruction. *Journal of Educational Psychology* 82 (2) pp 262-271

Rothbaum, F., Weisz, J.R. and Snyder, S.S. (1982) Changing the world and changing the self: A two-process model of perceived control. *Journal of Personality and Social Psychology* 42 pp 5-37

Seligman, M. E.P. (1975) *Helplessness: On Depression, Development and Death.* San Francisco: Freeman

Shain, D.D. and Kelliher, G. J. (1988) A study skills workshop as an integral part of orientation to medical school: The establishment of self-directed learning. *Proceedings of the Twenty-Seventh Annual Conference Research in Medical Education* Chicago, Il, Association of American Medical Colleges pp 91-96

Westfeldt, L. (1964) *F. Matthias Alexander: The Man and His Work*.Westport, CT: Associated Booksellers

Wilhite, S. C. (1990) Self-efficacy, locus of control, self-assessment of memory ability, and study activities as predictors of college course achievement. *Journal of Educational Psychology*, 82 (4) 696-700

Suggested Readings

Curley, R.B., Estrin, E.T., Thomas, J.W., and Rohwer, W.D., Jr. (1987) Relationships between study activities and achievement as a function of grade level and course characteristics. *Contemporary Educational Psychology*, 12, 324-343

Macan, T. H., Shahani, C., Dipboye, R. L., and Phillips, A. P. (1990) College students' time management: Correlations with academic performance and stress. *Journal of Educational Psychology*, 82 (4) 760-768

Marsh, H. W. (1990) Causal ordering of academic self-concept and academic achievement: A multiwave, longitudinal panel analysis. *Journal of Educational Psychology* 82 (4) 646-656

Reiser, M. F. (1984) *Mind, Brain, Body Toward a Convergence of Psychoanalysis and Neurobiology.* New York: Basic Books

Thomas, J.W., Iventosch, L., and Rohwer, W.D., Jr. (1987b) Relationships among student characteristics, study activities, and achievement as a function of course characteristics. *Contemporary Educational Psychology*, 12 pp 344-364

CHAPTER SEVEN • TEST-TAKING • DISCRIMINATION SKILLS

Taking tests may not be your favorite sport, but exams are a necessary part of your professional development. By the time you are ready to take the National Board Exam, you have traversed the rigorous path from naive medical student to competent, decision-making almost-professional. Your profession requires that you have the ability to make informed, rapid, and accurate decisions. By ruling out distractors and selecting correct answers in a test environment, you are developing the diagnostic skills you will need as a physician.

As a student, you may have been challenged by the prospect of gaining new information through study, but the reality of intellectual pursuits is that "all of society values the products of study rather than the process of knowledge acquisition" (Cohler, 1989). You have spent as much time studying as you were able to spend. You can't be more ready than you are right now. As you begin the examination challenge, you are on the road toward your goal--to become a physician!

Purpose

This chapter is designed to enhance your efficiency in decision-making through the use of specific test-taking techniques. These techniques include methods of attending to yourself, to the format of the exam, and to each exam question.

At the completion of this chapter, you will be able to accept the challenge of the exam with a positive attitude and sustain that attitude throughout the examination process. You will learn to analyze each examination question and read every aspect of the question thoroughly and carefully, so that you select the best answer. You will attend to your test environment, the equipment you need, the clothes to wear while taking the exam, and the care of your physical and emotional needs before and during the exam.

EQUIPMENT

- At least five or six not-too-sharp #2 pencils *

- Nonsmudge erasers

- Ear plugs

- Drinking water, chewing gum, or snacks

*In the past, you may have prepared yourself with freshly sharpened pencils to fill in your answer sheet. Sharp-tipped pencils require many strokes to fill in the answer blanks. If, instead, you use a fairly dull pencil, you will discover that the graphite spreads more easily, allowing you to proceed with greater speed.

THE EXAMINEE

You have taken apart, put together, and organized your basic science subjects. You have applied an organ system review of your material and dealt with your stress. You are ready to demonstrate your knowledge.

If you are like most students approaching an exam, you wish that you had more time to study. Of course you don't know everything there is to know, but you must convince yourself that you have studied thoroughly enough. You will have the rest of your life to learn more. But for now, trust your knowledge as it is, and be ready to follow your hunches as you work your way through the exam (Tryon, 1980).

Your mother was right when she told you to take care of yourself. Approach the exam as if you were an athlete. Attend to your basic physical and emotional needs. The most important success strategy you can develop is your ability to produce a good mood for the test. Clear your mind of extraneous thoughts. Get adequate sleep before the exam Take no drugs or medications that could compromise your thinking.

The evening before the exam, and the morning of the exam, eat well-balanced, high-protein meals. Do stress reduction exercises and deep-breathing exercises, relax your writing arm, and fortify yourself with positive self-talk.

Use any strategy that you can to increase constructive thoughts, reduce negative attitudes, increase efficiency, and reduce test anxiety. Look in the mirror and proudly proclaim your name with the prefix "Doctor." Can you hear yourself saying, "My name is Doctor . . . Go ahead, insert your first and last name after the word DOCTOR.

Dress for success. For some students, that means dressing in comfortable, loose-fitting clothing. For others, it means wearing clothes that make you feel professional. Often students report that when undue examination anxiety overtakes them, they can combat worry by dressing as if they were preparing to see patients. Once you are dressed like a physician, you can fool yourself into feeling like one.

Enter the examination room early so that you can select a seat in a well lighted, well ventilated, quiet location, free from distractions. Once you are seated, take a full belly breath and imagine yourself in the place you have conjured up in your "restful image" exercise. Imagine yourself receiving the successful results of the examination. See yourself celebrating your success. Now you are ready to begin the step-by-step, question and answer process of conquering the exam!

Prepare to screen out distractions. If the noise of sighs, page-turning, or chewing-gum popping disturbs you, you can improve your exam environment by wearing ear plugs. But be sure not to insert them until after you have heard any last-minute directions or announcements.

Take care of your physical comforts during the exam. If you know that you experience a dry mouth when you are under pressure, bring a bottle of water with you. If you are a gustatory type, prepare yourself with chewing gum or quiet and easy-to-access munchies. Raisins, pitted dates, shelled and unsalted nuts, cubes of cheese, carrot sticks, and beef jerky are a few of the favorites used by gustatory students.

If you are especially short or tall and are uncomfortable in the seats of the examination room, bring a back support or a small footstool with you so that you will not develop a distracting backache during the exam. If the overhead light bothers you, wear a cap with an eyeshade brim.

THE EXAM

Know the exam format. Spend a few moments looking through the exam pages. In leafing through, mark the top of the page that is at the one-quarter point, the half point, and the three-quarter point. How many questions are there? How much time do you have to answer all of the questions? In National Board examinations, figure that you have about 45 to 50 seconds for each question. Pace yourself.

In setting your pace, allow for time at the end to go back to rethink difficult items. Don't break your concentration. Discipline yourself not to look at the clock while you are reading a difficult question item. Like a racer who looks at the runners behind, this overattention to the clock will slow you down and rattle your confidence. There is plenty of time if you proceed systematically.

NBME question items are not ordered by degrees of difficulty or by subject area. The most difficult part of the NBME exam is the pacing and the variability of the exam. Therefore, you must make rapid adjustments as you move from item to item. Your best strategy is to answer the questions in the order in which they appear. Answer each question before you move on to the next. Proceed like a skillful detective, ready to ferret out the best option from a variety of possibilities.

Know the scoring rules. On NBME Part I examination, there is *no* penalty for guessing. Therefore it is to your advantage to answer *every* item. If you are clueless about an item, hazard a guess. Mark your test booklet with an "e.g." for an educated guess, and a "w.g." to indicate a wild guess. Mark your wild guess with the same letter each time.

Circle the number of the wild guess question on your test booklet and come back later to rethink this answer. By keeping your wild guesses consistent, you increase your statistical chances of hitting the right answer. And if, during the course of the exam, you think of a better answer, you will know just where to go to correct a wild guess.

Don't allow yourself to linger too long over a tough question. This will lower your confidence and may cause you to rush through answers on other questions that will be easier for you to answer later in the exam. Under no circumstances should you allow a tough question to contaminate your positive attitude as you move through the exam.

Examine each part of the stem and the answer choice to prevent too-hasty decisions. Make sure that you know what the emphasis of the stem is. Now be sure that your answer choice emphasizes the same thing. After reading the question stem, and before reading the answer alternatives, take a breath and allow a half second to think as you exhale.

Visualize the answer in your mind. Then look for this answer among the choices offered. This is especially helpful for **Perceiving** types who tend to talk themselves into wrong answers, and for **Judgers** who answer too quickly (Shain, 1989). Make use of partial information to draw inferences when the answer alternative seems unclear. Drawing inferences is what you will do as a professional diagnostician; therefore, the exam helps accustom you to that practice.

Read *all* of the possible choices even if you think the first or second choice is correct. **Judging** types take heed. Test writers like to put their best distractors in the first or second position to catch the unsuspecting, hasty examinee.

Optimal answer selection requires skill in blocking out distractions from among the variety of answer choices. To block out distractors, you will need to mark the stem of the question and the answer choices as you move through the questions. Simplify answer possibilities by saying "yes," "no," or "not sure" to the alternatives. Always record your answer choice in writing. Place a "T" (yes) or "F" (no) or "?" (not sure) next to each answer possibility.

Beware of reading too much into a question. Unless otherwise specified, in items that ask for the *cause* in the stem and the *result* in the answer alternative, remember to choose the alternative that is most *directly* related to the effect described. For example, in the steps of a process in which A leads to B, which leads to C, which leads to D, if the stem asks what causes D, your best choice would most likely be C, *not* A.

Take the time to read and interpret the question carefully. If two answer alternatives overlap or have essentially the same meaning, both are probably correct if, and only if, the format allows for more than one correct answer. Both are most likely incorrect if the format allows for only one correct statement. Underline significant words in the question stem. Be sure to mark special qualifying words, e.g., "especially" or negative words, such as "except," "least likely," and "will not exhibit." Circle the verb. Make a chart or diagram of the directions.

One Best Answer--Positive Stem

The one-best-answer format is the most frequently used multiple-choice question. The question stem consists of: either a partial statement, a direct question, or a single word followed by several (usually five) answer choices. Although several of the answer choices may appear correct, only one includes the most *specific* answer for the question, and is therefore the BEST answer choice. Proceed through the answer choices marking each one "T," "F," or "?" as you go.

Eliminate those alternatives that may be plausible but are less appropriate. As you read the answer possibilities, circle words that are repeated in two or more of the answer alternatives; this circling process will help you to focus on the point of the item.

Let's answer the following one-best-answer type taken from page 81 of the Oklahoma Notes *Neuroanatomy* book:

6. A <u>unilateral lesion</u> of the <u>internal</u> capsule involving the <u>genu and the posterior limb</u> would cause:

       E

F   A. Contralateral <u>total</u> facial paralysis.

     B. Contralateral limb paralysis and ipsilateral lower facial paralysis.

F   C. Ipsilateral limb paralysis and ipsilateral lower facial paralysis.

     D. Contralateral limb paralysis and contralateral lower facial paralysis.

?   E. Ipsilateral total facial paralysis and contralateral limb paralysis.

There is no substitute for knowing your material. But if you don't, or you can't remember, there are ways to use the information presented to make an educated guess.

Notice the similarity between answers B and D. Both include the phrases *Contralateral limb paralysis* and *lower facial paralysis*. If I were forced to venture a guess, because I know that ipsilateral limb paralysis is false, I would probably choose B or D because they share two variables. As it happens, the answer is D.

One Best Answer--Negative Stem

In the case of the negative stem, you will need to switch from positive to negative thinking. In order to avoid confusion, you will simplify your thinking if you follow these steps:

- circle the negative word in the stem

- omit the negative word and read the stem as a positive statement

- mark each alternative T, F, or ? as you go through your answer

  options.

Let's apply this system by using the following example taken from page 224 of the Oklahoma Notes *Pathology* book:

14. Manifestations of <u>right-sided heart failure</u> might include all of the following

     A. Ascites.

     B. Hepatic congestion.

     C. Pulmonary edema.

     D. Splenomegaly.

Take out the negative word. Read the question in the affirmative, and proceed to answer, marking the T, F, and ?.

Manifestations of <u>right-sided heart failure</u> might include all of the following:

   ?   A.   Ascites.

   T   B. Hepatic congestion.

   F   C. <u>Pulmonary edema.</u>

   T   D. Splenomegaly.

Now select the only F answer (in this case it is C) and mark the corresponding letter as your answer. Again, you can take advantage of partial information. The fact that you were not sure about A and marked it with a question mark doesn't matter, since you are *sure* that C is False.

When you proceed logically and carefully, you can allow yourself to use partial information or to follow your hunches to arrive at the correct answer.

Matching-Type Questions

The important feature of matching-type questions is that they test your ability to distinguish among closely related items such as diseases, conditions, drugs, signs, symptoms, or structures.

Each group of matching-type questions consists of lettered headings, a diagram, or a table with several components followed by a list of numbered words, statements, or phrases. You are asked to select the one lettered heading or lettered component that is most closely associated with the numbered item. Each lettered heading or lettered component may be selected once, more than once, or not at all.

Read the question stem, underline the important feature being emphasized in the question, and then ask yourself about the association *before* looking at the answer possibilities.

To avoid becoming confused by the answer possibilities, some students find it helpful to make a chart of answer possibilities in the margin to the left of the questions.

Let's try a question taken from page 226 of the Oklahoma Notes *Microbiology and Immunology* book.

Match the antigen used in serologic diagnosis in the right hand column with the disease listed in the left hand column. An answer may be used more than once or not at all.

83. Cryptoccal meningitis

84. Haemophilus meningitis

85. Poliomyelitis

A. Erythrocytes

B. Viable bacteria

C. Viable viruses

D. Capsular antigens

E. Attenuated protozoa

See if the question stems on the left have anything in common. Underline the qualifying words. Notice the importance of keeping your focus on the items in the left-hand column. The unrelated answer choices on the right can distract you if you read them first.

Now make your chart in the left margin and underline your answer choice as follows.

A. B. C. _D._ E. __ 83. Cryptoccal meningitis

A. B. C. _D._ E __ 84. Haemophilus meningitis

A. B. _C._ D. E __ 85. Poliomyelitis

A. Erythrocytes

B. Viable bacteria

C. Viable viruses

D. Capsular antigens

E. Attenuated protozoa

How did you reach the correct answer? Did you notice that 83 and 84 had anything in common? Is that why the answer for both is _D_?

Case History Type Questions

Because case history questions test the examinee's problem-solving capabilities, they are appearing more on current National Boards. The case history consists of a clinical situation, followed by a series of questions pertaining to the case. Analyze each part of the case history, and select the best answer.

When reading a case history, label the sections of the case in the margin. Mark transition points with a double slash mark (//). In that way, when a question is asked, you will be able to go directly to the specific part of the history that applies to the question.

Typical labels for case histories are: *History, Signs and Symptoms, Lab Findings (LbF), Treatment (Rx), Diagnosis (Dx), Prognosis, Outcome.* Let's label and insert // marks in the following example of a case history question:

(Hist)   A 65 year-old surgeon was in good health except for a nine-year history

(LbF)   of diabetes mellitus and hypertension (blood pressure of 160/94 mm Hg).// He

(Sgns)   experienced severe crushing pericardial pain while shoveling snow. He collapsed

    and was rushed to the hospital // where he was found to be in shock, cyanotic with

(Sym)   hypotension and a rapid, weak pulse. The patient was given oxygen and supportive

(Rx)   therapy. He showed improvement. His blood pressure returned to its

(Result) previous level.// Seven days after admission, after a bowel movement, the

(Dx)   patient died suddenly.// Found at autopsy was extensive myocardial infarction.

The essay or story portion of the question above will be followed by a series of questions related to: direct cause of death, laboratory findings of the renal system related to the diabetes mellitus, histological features of the original infarct, and pathological features of the cardiac muscle based on the hypertension and the patient's condition. In order to find your way back through the material, you will need to take the time to label the separate and distinct parts of the history, as we have above.

Often students overlook the tricky, seemingly unrelated aspects of the question, such as age, sex, and occupation. In this case, the fact that the patient was a surgeon indicates that he had access to health care and was socially and economically advantaged. His age, symptoms, treatment, and diagnosis will be important aspects of reasoning through your answers in this question.

K-Type Format

Although National Board exams have dropped the K-type format, many classroom shelf exams retain that pattern of multiple-choice questions. Should you confront the K-type format, you will see the following instructions:

For each of the incomplete statements, one or more of the completions given is correct.

The answer is

A. if only (1), (2), and (3) are correct.

B. if only (1) and (3) are correct.

C. if only (2) and (4) are correct.

D. if only (4) is correct.

E. if all are correct.

Make a chart of the possible answers and rewrite the directions as follows:

$$A= T, T, T, F$$
$$B= T, F, T, F$$
$$C= F, T, F, T$$
$$D= F, F, F, T$$
$$E= T, T, T, T$$

In the answer chart above, you may have noticed that the answers in the 1 and 3 position have something in common. If answer alternative 1 is correct, so will answer choice 3 be correct. If answer alternative 1 is false, 3 will also be false. How do you know that? Because the directions tell you so. Therefore, reading both 1 and 3 becomes an unnecessary use of time.

The best way to save time when answering K-type questions is to read the answer alternatives in this order: read 4, then 2, then either 1 or 3, whichever is shorter.

Proceed to answer the K-types with your pencil in hand, marking the *T*, *F*, or *?* answers along the margin side of the answer alternatives as you go.

Let's practice by using an example taken from page 116 of the Oklahoma Notes *Microbiology and Immunology:*

For each of the incomplete statements, one or more of the completions given is correct. The answer is

A. if only (1), (2), and (3) are correct.

B. if only (1) and (3) are correct.

C. if only (2) and (4) are correct.

D. if only (4) is correct.

E. if all are correct.

Again, rewrite the directions: A= T, T, T, F

B= T, F, T, F

C= F, T, F, T

D= F, F, F, T

E= T, T, T, T

Once your directions are clear, move on to the question:

Infections are a significant cause of death in patients with

T   1. Bruton's hypogammaglobulemia.

T   2. Di George syndrome.

T   3. chromic granulomatous disease.

T   4. systemic lupus erythematosus.

If you didn't remember what Bruton's disease was but you did know that answer 3 was correct, you would know that 1 must also be correct. Therefore, because all answer options are true, the answer is E.

Question Analysis

Always separate the components of the question into phrases to which you can say yes (T) or no (F) or don't know (?). When you break down the question into phrases and consider each phrase as a separate question, you will feel in control of the data. Certain that each part of your answer is correct, through this thorough approach you will be enabled to maintain composure and proceed with confidence. As you look at the next K-type question, break the answer choices into phrases, marking each with *T, F*, or *?* as you go through the question.

The question as it is written reads:

The semilunar valves

1. are characterized by the presence of papillary muscles and chordae tendinae

2. are the outflow valves of the heart, and are located between the right ventricle and the

   pulmonary trunk, and the left ventricle and the aorta.

3. close as a result of the contraction of cardiac muscle anchored to the base of the valve and

   to the cardiac skeleton.

4. function to prevent the reflux of blood into the ventricles during ventricular relaxation.

Read the question stem again. Then underline what is being asked. The label words *function, location, results* that you wrote in your notes will jump out at you.

Let's follow each phrase step by step. Insert lines between the question phrases. Write a *T* or an *F* above each section of the question; then, place a *T* or an *F* in the margin. Start with answer option 4, then go to 2, then either 1 or 3, whichever is shorter.

The <u>semilunar</u> valves

F 1. are <u>characterized</u> by the presence of papillary muscles // and chordae tendinae.

T 2. are the <u>outflow</u> valves of the heart, // and are <u>located</u> between the

   right ventricle and the pulmonary trunk, // and the *left* ventricle and the *aorta*.

F 3. close as a result of <u>*contraction*</u> of cardiac muscle // <u>anchored</u>

   to the *base* of the valve // and to the *cardiac skeleton*.

T 4. function to *prevent* the <u>reflux of blood</u> // into the *ventricle*// during

   ventricular *relaxation*.

Once I answered that 4 and 2 are correct, I read the first phrase of answer choice 1, and knew that *characterized by the presence of papillary muscles* was false. I no longer had to read any more of answer option 1 or 3, and marked answer *C*. Using a phrase-by-phrase approach will ensure accuracy and save time.

THREE STEPS IN THE IF-ALL-ELSE-FAILS DEPARTMENT

Memory Jogs by Content Recall

Difficult and unanswered questions can be upsetting. Reset your mood, and regain control. If you feel baffled by a question, use the following recall techniques.

Ask yourself: *What keeps me from answering this question?*

- Do I understand the language of the question?
- Did I pay attention to the verbs so I am sure I know what are they asking?
- Did I break the phrases of the question into parts. Did I stop to notice the commas?
- Did I mark a *T* or *F* above each phrase of the question?
- Did I diagram the process mentioned in the stem?
- Did I make a sketch of the identified structure?
- Before reading the answer options, did I summarize the question in my own words?
- Did I think about the relationship of structure, function, and mechanism of action as they relate to the question?

Memory Jogs by Study Situation Context Recall

If you understand the question but cannot recall the answer, probe your memory by recreating the circumstances in which you learned the information.

Think about the professor's voice when she lectured about this material. Where were you sitting?

Picture your notes. When you studied this subject, what color did you use to highlight or to label your notes?

What music did you hear while studying this information?

What were you doing immediately before and after you studied this material?

Memory Jogs by Material Context Recall

If contextual memory probing fails, ask yourself organizational questions about the material itself. Is what you are trying to remember a part of something else?

Ask: *Does X have some subtopics I can remember? What is the relationship between X and Y? What is an analogy to X? Does X lead to something else?*

Did another question on the exam give you a clue? If not, guess, and move on.

GUESSING AND ANALYZING

Your first-guess answer is the one that comes from somewhere in the deep recesses of your unconscious memory bank: therefore, the first-guess answer has a high likelihood of being correct. Change the first-guess answer *only* when you can think of an obvious, concrete reason that proves your first choice wrong.

When you are anxious, feeling emotionally vulnerable, or overtired, you will have a tendency to second-guess yourself into wrong answers (Wilhite, 1990). If you *think* something is false when you first read it, then trust that it *is* false. Fancy-sounding false answers are inserted into examinations to test your ability to resist seductively complex distractions.

Although guessing can make you uncomfortable, remember: DO NOT LEAVE ANY ANSWER BLANK.

If you are making a *wild guess*, remember to mark *w.g* in the margin of your test booklet and move on. If you are making an educated guess, mark an *e.g.* in the margin.

Wrong answers are opportunities for increased learning. All exams help you discover what you need to review. If you really want to cement material in your brain forever, go back after an exam, and figure out why it is you missed a particular question.

To become your own educational diagnostician, use the Performance Analysis--Test- Taking chart on the following page.

PERFORMANCE ANALYSIS--TEST-TAKING

Subject_____

Directions: Look through the questions you missed. Using the 17 categories listed below, identify the primary factors for your error. Label each incorrect item with the corresponding number. Tally each factor in the chart at the bottom of the page. Write your strategies for avoiding the same mistakes next time.

1. I did not know the facts or couldn't remember them.

2. I simply did not study long enough.

3. I did not read all of the options carefully; I chose the first one that sounded right.

4. I failed to consider key words such as : *except, least likely, mostly, always*

5. I read too much into the question, got bogged down, and missed the main point.

6. I did not think through the logic of the question.

7. I changed the answer. My first response was correct.

8. Vocabulary was a problem.

9. I read part of the question stem and took the rest for granted.

10. I did not finish in the time allotted and had to do some wild guessing at the end.

11. I did not work through the process of elimination in selecting the best answer.

12. I failed to recognize relationships of concepts such as Function, Structure, and Mechanism of Action.

13. I failed to recognize compare/contrast data.

14. I failed to recognize clinical implications.

15. I had difficulty with simple recall.

16. I had difficulty with details.

17. I had difficulty with concepts.

1	2	3	4	5	6	7	8	9	10	11	12	13	14	15	16	17

Future Corrective Strategies:

SUMMARY

You are ready to demonstrate the results of your study efforts. Set your mind to the exciting challenge. Gather your not-too-sharp pencils in hand. Have your ear plugs ready to block out the noise. Take a deep breath, and get ready to congratulate yourself on a job well done! You will if you remember to:

1. keep a positive attitude

2. take care of your physical and emotional needs before, during, and after the exam

3. know the format of the exam

4. know the overall time allotted. Proceed with the test at a careful, deliberate, steady pace. Avoid spending too much time on any one question.

5. approach disturbing questions as a memory contest. If you are stumped, fill in your best guess and move on with a promise to return to it later. Don't compromise your success by concentrating on a likely loser, thereby jeopardizing several winners because you ran out of time. Remember that the next question may be your opportunity to feel confident again.

6. allow time to review your answers. Be sure that you do not skip a question, fail to read through all the choices, or misinterpret a question.

7. DO NOT CHANGE AN ANSWER unless there is a very good reason for doing so. Unless you have misread the question, your first choice is usually correct. When you review your guesses, change your answer if, and *only* if:

   • you have additional information

   • you may have overlooked qualifying words such as *except, least likely*, etc.

   • you failed to read the stem or any part of the question correctly.

8. read each phrase of the question, stop and mark *T* or *F* above each phrase.

9. take time to label case history questions.

You are in control of yourself, the material, and your results. Go to it doctor-to-be!

References:

Cohler, B. (1989) Psychoanalysis and education: Motive, meaning, and self. In *Learning and Education: Psychoanalytic Perspectives,* Field, K., Cohler, B. and Wool, G. Editors Madison, CT: International Universities Press Inc, pp 11-68

Shain, D. D. (1989) Self-directed learning and collegial interaction through the use of the Myers-Briggs Type Indicator in medical education. In *Proceedings APT VIII Biennial International Conference, Boulder CO Frontiers of Psychological Type* Gainsville, FL Association for Psychological Type pp 101-104

Tryon, G.B. (1980) The measurement and treatment of test anxiety. *Review of Educational Research* 50 pp 343-372

Wilhite, S. C. (1990) Self-efficacy, locus of control, self-assessment of memory ability, and study activities as predictors of college course achievement. *Journal of Educational Psychology,* 82 (4) pp 696-700

Suggested readings

Marton, F. and Saljo, R. (1976) On qualitative differences in learning II -- Outcomes as a function of the learner's conception of the task. *British Journal of Educational Psychology* 46 pp 233-243

Shain, D.D. and Kelliher, G.J. (1987) Reduction of resource use through the provision of a prematriculation program. *Innovations in Medical Education* Wash., D.C. 98th Annual Meeting of the American Medical Association

CHAPTER EIGHT • ORGANIZING AND WORKING IN A STUDY GROUP

Studying is usually a solitary activity. Once you have established what you know and identified what you don't know, a study group is a dynamic place to deepen understanding, correct misconceptions, and practice collegial communication and consultation skills. Students who spend at least two hours weekly in *well-organized* study groups have found the experience invaluable as preparation for examinations and for professional consultations (Leon and Martinez, 1989; Shain and Kelliher, 1988).

The stimulation of colleagues' questions and discussion, and the encouragement of the group, can spur you on and help you to overcome subject phobias and weaknesses. When you teach their colleagues, the group teaching experience clarifies facts and helps you to integrate related material. Through teaching, you become active and use all of your perceptual possibilities--in group, you see, say, write, analyze, synthesize, and reinforce your learning.

In the past, you may have experienced study groups as time-wasters. More than likely that was because the group was neither well focused nor properly organized. Groups that deteriorate into social gatherings usually do so because the members are unskilled in group dynamics (Hare et al.,1955).

Purpose

This chapter will provide guidelines for establishing and using time-conserving study groups. Methods for selecting group members, setting up agendas, establishing contracts for procedures, individual responsibility, and study content will be presented.

SOME DOS AND DON'TS OF GROUPS

Do Establish Structure

- Group membership. Numbers should be limited to no more than five or six colleagues of a variety of complementary types. (**ES** and **EN**, **IS** and **IN** . . .) Group members need not be those folks with whom you socialize. In fact, the more professional and the less personal you can keep the group, the better.

- Agenda. Members must decide in advance of the group meeting on a realistic, achievable agenda.

- Time and place. The group should meet in twice-weekly, two-hour sessions. Meeting time and place should be the same each week.

- Leadership. In order to stay focused on the study tasks and to prevent the time-consuming distractions of undue socialization, the group should appoint a permanent or a rotating convener who will keep the group on target during the study session. A rotating or permanent scribe should keep notes of the discussion. To reinforce the memory curve, notes should be photocopied and distributed to all group members within 24 hours of the group meeting (see Chapter Two • Time Management and Memory).

- Content. Content must be specific and comments limited to the subject matter.

- Accountability. Each member of the group must be accountable to the others. Members must have specific tasks to perform before, during, and after the meeting. Everyone should participate in the group discussion. Rules for attendance, punctuality, and confidentiality must be made explicit, and the consequences for breaking the rules must be discussed openly.

- Emotional climate and ground rules. Group process is enhanced when members use the group to reinforce a positive self-image for each group member.

Don't Get Sloppy

- Don't allow yourself or any member of the group to attend unprepared.

- Don't allow group meetings to become rap sessions.

- Don't allow yourself or anyone else to break the rules.

- Don't allow complaining to take up group time. Negative comments such as: *I can't believe your question* . . . or critical behind-the-back talk or chit-chat should not be permitted.

GROUP STUDY TASKS • ORGAN SYSTEM REVIEW

An organ system review is especially amenable to group discussion. For group procedure to be time-efficient and valuable, group members should follow a structured content format. The following steps for study-group-effective activity have worked in medical schools in the U.S.A., Mexico, and Puerto Rico.

Choosing the Study Focus

As in the subject-by-subject Board Review study method described in Chapter Five • Preparing for National Board Examinations, your chosen study areas should be those that gave you difficulty in the past. For example, if you had trouble with physiology and if the diseases and functioning of the kidney were unclear when you first encountered them, you will volunteer to be the group expert on renal physiology. Work through all aspects of the organ system thoroughly. When that organ system is learned, work through other weak areas in the same way.

Preparation

Read alone in your weakest subject area and develop a matrix of at least five questions combining structure, function, mechanism of action, requirements for the mechanism of action, and results in terms of cause and effect. Come to group prepared to ask and discuss your questions.

Become an Expert

Build an organ system/pathology question matrix based on the model shown in Chapter Five. Prepare for group discussion by researching your questions as much as you are able. Your structured question matrix, your areas of newly acquired expertise, and those areas that you are unsure about will become the impetus for group discussion. Armed with your identified deficits, you will lead the discussion, asking the group to challenge you with their questions.

Follow Group Rules

Agree to twice-weekly, two-hour sessions and adhere to the agenda. Don't be afraid to ask others to stay focused on the topic and stick to the rules.

Reveal Your Weaknesses

Remember that you will *not* use the group to demonstrate your strengths. You already have those in tow. The group is there for you to overcome your deficiencies. Once you have been able to identify your weak areas for yourself, the process of formulating questions about uncertain areas will help you to reach clarity. By verbalizing your confusions, concerns, and anxieties, you allow the group to direct you toward relevant questions and further study. In group, you master your shortcomings, meet your study tasks directly, and ready yourself for the challenge of the written exam.

APPLICATION OF THE PROBLEM-SOLVING MODEL TO GROUPS

We usually solve our problems alone. However, in study groups, case conferences, and consultations with other professionals we need to work with colleagues to solve problems. Problem-solving in a group takes practice (McCaulley, 1987).

When working in problem-solving groups, each member will need to define the problem as described in Chapter Four • Problem-Solving. Each individual must be responsible for establishing achievable goals. The group must agree to seek consensus and closure, or to allow for differences to remain unresolved. All members of a problem-solving group can make valuable contributions. The learning style gifts of each member of the group should be used in turn.

For time-efficient group discussion, first ask the **Sensors** to describe all of the details available in the present. Next ask the **Intuitives** to develop hypotheses and examine and explore the possible future consequences of any aspect of the problem solution. Then the **Thinkers** should make their critical, objective analysis of the tasks that have been accomplished, and finally the **Feelers** should use their talents to tend to the group dynamics and discuss the relative value of the data, hypothesis, and steps that have been taken toward the solution of the problem.

As members contribute to the discussion, they should remained focused and follow the problem-solving steps delineated above. Problem definition, strategy formulation, subgoal construction, execution of the strategy, and evaluation of progress can provide a productive use of the group's talents in a problem-solving session.

References

Hare, A. P., Borgatta, E. F., Bales, R. F.,Editors. (1955) *Small Groups: Studies In Social Interaction.* New York: Alfred A. Knopf

Leon, R. and Martinez, F. (1989) Recent developments in medical education at the Universidad Autonoma De Guadalajara School Of Medicine. Wash., D.C. Innovations in Medical Education, American Association of Medical Colleges

McCaulley, M. H. (1987) *Developing Critical Thinking and Problem-Solving Abilities: New Directions for Teaching and Learning* San Francisco: Jossey-Bass

Shain, D.D. and Kelliher, G.J. (1987) Reduction of resource use through the provision of a prematriculation program. *Innovations in Medical Education* Wash., D.C. 98th Annual Meeting of the American Medical Association

Suggested Readings

Goffman, E. (1967) *Interaction Ritual: Essays in Face-to-Face Behavior.* Chicago: Aldine Publishing Co.

Pollak, G. (1975) *Leadership of Discussion Groups; Case Material and Theory.* New York: Spectrum Publications

Shain, D. D. (1989) Self-directed learning and collegial interaction through the use of the Myers-Briggs Type Indicator in medical education In *Proceedings APT VIII Biennial International Conference, Boulder CO Frontiers of Psychological Type* Gainsville, FL Association for Psychological Type pp 101-104